Lymphedema Self-Care Manual

4th edition

Phyllis Tubbs-Gingerich, RN,BSN,LE, CLT
Lymphedema Specialist
Board Certified Mastectomy Fitter
Medical Esthetician
Certified Gradient Compression Designer/Fitter

Lymphedema Self-Care Manual ©
Published by FufiKing Publishing Company
Printed: 4th edition June, 2022

Acknowledgments

A *Big* Thank-You To:

Patients — without their input, this manual would not be possible

Our suppliers and fabricators

All our supporters throughout 32 years' service

Bill King, EdD — editing & technical assistance

Daniel Miranda — editing & technical assistance

Forward

Lymphedema is a life-changing, chronic condition that affects an estimated 250 million people worldwide. Thus, the need for a detailed resource guide for lymphedema self-care prompted the publication of this "easy-to-carry" manual. We hope our revised 4th edition will be more detailed in answering questions you have about lymphedema and will guide you through a better understanding of self-care.

The best way to treat lymphedema is to:
- Get as much information as possible about lymphedema.
- Seek proper care and instructions from a bona fide lymphedema specialist.
- Secure materials and supplies necessary to properly maintain lymphedema.

This book is not intended to be a medical manual or to replace your physician's care and advice. It should serve as a guide to aid in self-care and maintenance of lymphedema, skin and wound care. It is the culmination of over 40 years' experience in the field of cancer, lymphedema, skin and wound care. Self-care suggestions in this book are the direct result of patients' subjective comments, which prompted us to research better methods of treatment. Over the years these formulas have been used in treating our patients, and have not only become part of our clinic's protocol for therapy, but have proven to be a vital tool for education of patients in self care and maintenance. This constant exchange of information between patient and care-giver continues to be the basis for individualized patient care at our clinic.

Table of Contents

Chapter 10 - Miscellaneous Information

Introduction

The Lymphatic System — is primarily comprised of **lymphatic vessels** (lymphatics), **lymph nodes,** and **lymph**. The lymphatic system is an important part of the body's immune system because lymphatics transport lymph, which contains *macrophages* (white blood cells that kill bacteria and clean up cellular wastes), as well as antibodies and other protein substances that fight infection. Also contained in the lymph are water and waste materials consisting of chemical, organic, and inorganic body cell products, as well as cell residue, including foreign organisms like viruses and bacteria.

The lymphatic system as the "garbage system of the body," is a one-way system eliminating wastes produced by working body cells and carrying these wastes to excretory organs for elimination, primarily by the kidneys. However, it has been our experience that in cases of chronic (long-term) lymphedema with *fibrosis* (hardening and congestion of tissues), waste products are also being eliminated by means of other excretory organs: pores of the skin, exhalation of the lungs, and bowel movements. During intensive combined decongestive therapy for lymphedema, patients have reported very pungent odorous perspiration, especially in the armpits (axilla) and groin, bad breath, and foul-smelling bowel movements.

Lymph — is the clear, yellowish, slightly sticky liquid that flows from an open wound after bleeding ceases. It is the fluid that "bathes" all our body cells and keeps body tissues moist. Lymph is manufactured by the body – the result of the breakdown of food and liquids we have eaten that is absorbed by the small intestines and transported to all parts of the body ("you are what you eat"). Lymph contains cellular protein debris, microorganisms, bacteria, body cell wastes, and other waste particles too large for the veins to transport. Only the lymphatics have the capacity to transport these larger particles for elimination. Lymph must be in a constant state of movement or it will stagnate and become more thickened, causing severe side effects, e.g., *fibrosis,* infection, pain, heaviness, immobility, and cellulitis (infection of the skin and underlying tissues). When *fibrosis* occurs in the tissues, lymph fluid below the affected area cannot pass through, leaving the entire area prone to infection and cellulitis. In addition, thickened lymph in the joints "lock up" the joints, decreasing movement, flexibility, and producing pain. In fact, patients with lymphedema have reported that swelling due to an increase of lymph fluid and waste products in an affected area has produced greater levels of discomfort in not only the joints but also the tissues. Since lymph contains body waste products, it is essential that anyone caring for a lymphedema patient, including the patient, should carefully wash hands before making contact with an affected lymphedematous area. Patients with lymphedema are much more prone to infections.

Lymphatics are tubes or vessels that transport lymph from all parts of the body for elimination. The lymphatic tubes (lumen) have small, muscular, pump-like chambers which automatically move lymph through smaller lymphatic channels into larger lymphatic channels. When the body is at rest, lymph moves progressively through lymphatics (lymph vessels) at a rate of approximately 7x/ minute. Dur-ing exercise, movement of lymph increases dramatically. Only lymphatic vessels have the capacity to transport larger cell debris and other protein waste particles found in lymph. In a healthy state, lymphatics are designed and equipped to transport 10% of all body fluids containing wastes — the veins transport 90%. When this 90/10 equation is disrupted, fluids back up, causing swelling. Forty percent (40%) of all lymphatics in the body are just under the surface of the skin. Therefore, manual lymph drainage focuses on stimulating the smaller lymphatics in this space called the "ground substance" (connective tissue), moving lymph into collateral lymphatic pathways and by-passing areas of congestion.

Lymph Nodes — Important to the immune system, the **primary function** of these kidney-shaped organs is to filter out impurities, concentrate lymph, and store white blood cells (lymphocytes) which kill viruses and bacteria.

There are about 600-900 lymph nodes in the human body, depending upon each person's size and body build. About 200-300 lymph nodes are located in the neck, and the remaining lymph nodes are distributed throughout strategic areas of the body: the armpits (axilla), the groins (inguinals), along the spinal column, and approximately 100-200 lymph nodes lining the bowel and intestines.

The Lymphatic System

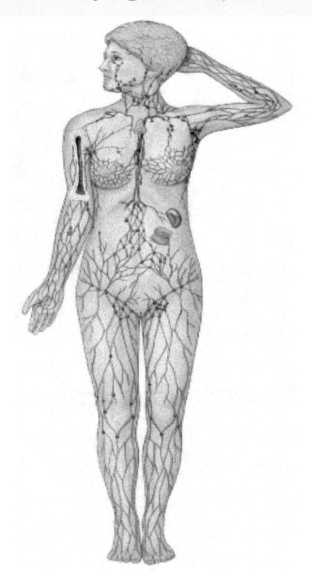

Lymphatic System - Arm

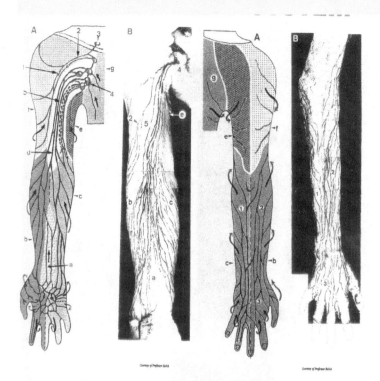

Courtesy of Professor Rabb

Courtesy of Professor Rabb

Lymphatic bundles and lymphatic territories on the upper extremity (anterior)

A. graphic description
B. corpse
a) medial forearm bundle
b) radial forearm bundle
c) ulnar forearm bundle
d) medial upper arm territory
e) dorso-medial upper arm territory
f) dorso-lateral upper arm and shoulder territory
g) upper trunk quadrant
1. deltoid-pectoral lymph nodes
2. deltoid bundle
3. supraclavicular lymph nodes
4. axillary lymph nodes
5. medial upper arm bundle

Lymphatic bundles and lymphatic territories on the upper extremity (posterior)

A. graphic description
B. corpse
1. ulnar forearm bundle
2. radial forearm bundle
3. anastomosis between 1 & 2
b) radial territory
c) ulnar territory
e) dorso-medial upper arm territory
f) dorso-lateral upper arm territory
g) upper trunk quadrant

Lymphatics of Head

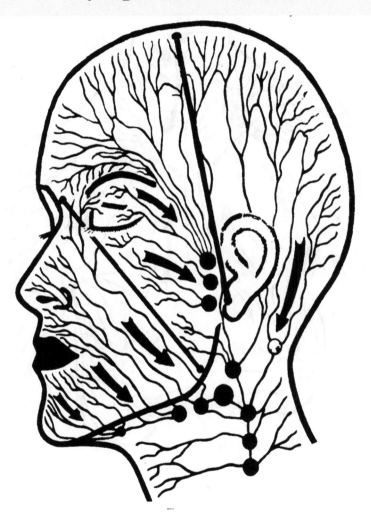

Breast & Upper Torso

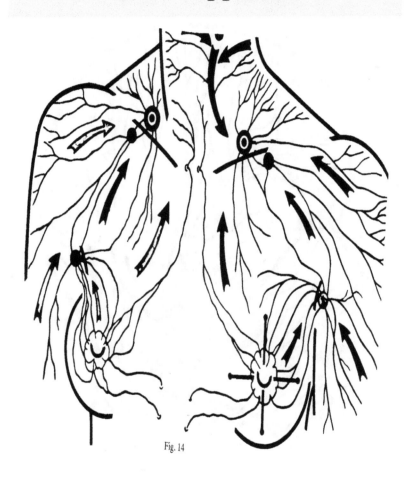

Fig. 14

Anterior Trunk Lymphatics

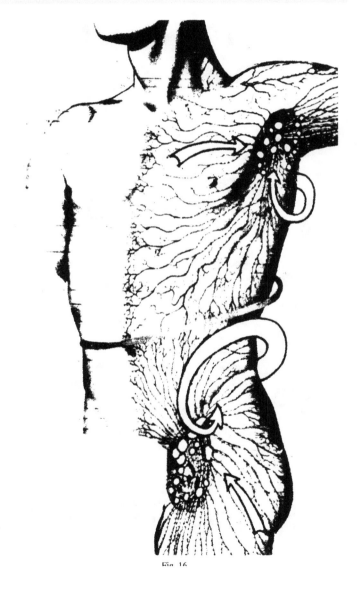

Fig. 16

Posterior Trunk Lymphatics

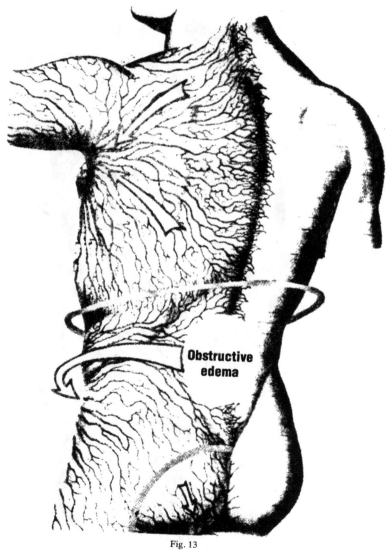

Obstructive edema

Fig. 13

Lymphatic System - Legs

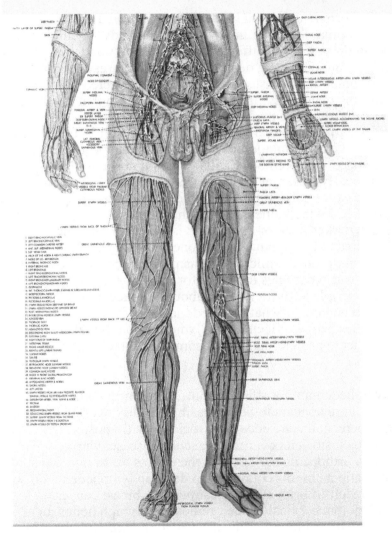

Chapter 1

Lymphedema

"The chronic unknown hidden disease," can affect any man, woman, or child in any part of the body — children being most severely affected. When lymph nodes or lymph vessels are damaged, destroyed, or missing resulting in an accumulation of wastes and fluids in an affected body part, swelling occurs. Lymphedema is a condition that results in the breakdown of the body's ability to remove and filter *intercellular* (between cells) fluids. The result is an excessive accumulation of *lymph* (fluid that originates in the spaces between body cells). Lymph normally flows into a successively larger series of vessels deeper in the body and is eventually emptied into the venous system and excreted by the kidneys. When this occurs, the urine will be much darker in color and more viscous in consistency. Hundreds of lymph nodes stationed throughout the body filter out proteins, micro-organisms, body cell wastes, and other waste particles too large for the veins to transport. Most people know very little about lymphedema, how and why it occurs, or what can be done about it. This not only includes people affected with lymphedema, but also those healthcare professionals who come in contact with the disease.

Lymphedema now affects about 2% of our population, and this figure appears to be increasing steadily. Not included in this percentage are edemas associated with: post surgery, venous insufficiency, cardiovascular disease, varicose veins, orthopedic surgery and the effects of trauma. Most of the patients in this country who develop lymphedema do so as a result of prior cancer treatment for breast cancer, melanoma, cervical cancer, removal of lymph nodes, or radiation for tumors. This is *secondary lymphedema*. The most extreme form of secondary lymphedema is elephantiasis. Elephantiasis is characterized by tremendous swelling,

21

and the overlying skin is very dark in color, thick, and coarse, and appears very similar to elephant skin in texture. This condition can develop after long periods of untreated lymphedema. Still other cases of lymphedema develop as a result of burns, trauma from surgery, accidents, cuts or breaks in the skin, or even insect bites. There are also large numbers of patients who are born with this condition, which is *primary lymphedema.*

As patients and care givers, you know how difficult it has been to not only get information about lymphedema but also to find bona fide lymphedema treatment. Very little in the way of therapy has been available to relieve both the physical and emotional distress brought on by this condition. One of the problems of lymphedema is that it does not remain stationary – it continually progresses and changes. Untreated lymphedema can result in grossly swollen body parts containing areas of stagnated lymph leading to fibrosis. Because this fluid is protein-rich, it is a perfect medium for growth of bacteria and the area/limb becomes highly susceptible to infection and cellulitis. Any break in the skin can open the way for bacteria to enter. Furthermore, severe swelling and fibrosis leads to immobility due to increased swelling in the joints, chronic infections because of stagnation of wastes in the tissues of the affected part, irreversible complications and a cancer known as *lymphangiosarcoma.* And, since lymphedema is a chronic disease, it requires proper treatment and maintenance to control swelling, prevent complications, and increase quality of life. The most severely affected are children with primary lymphedema. Most of these have an accompanying congenital condition known as *Klippel-Trenaunay*, which not only affects body tissues, but also blood vessels and bones.The resulting effects are port wine stains with severe varicose veins, swollen bulbous tissues, especially of the feet and toes, and unequal bone growth of the legs. Since each lymphedema case is different, these children, as well as all lymphedema patients, must be treated individually or case specific.

How Lymphedema Develops

When lymph nodes or lymphatics are destroyed, damaged or obstructed, lymph seeps out into the tissues, but the lymphatic capillaries do not let much fluid back in. Water and *macrophages* (proteins and other larger particles) accumulate in the tissues. If left untreated, eventually the swelling becomes so severe, the entire area/limb is distended and distorted. The presence of proteins and *macrophages* can trigger a chronic inflammatory reaction, which over time, can produce changes in the tissues involved. In the early stages of lymphedema, the swollen area is soft and becomes pitted when pressed ("pitting edema"). As the condition advances, the chronic inflammation and oxygen deprivation causes the tissues to become more *fibrous* (thread-like, woodsy), the skin to grow dry and hard (*fibrotic*) and the tissues no longer yield to pressure. When fibrosis occurs, lymph cannot pass beyond or through this area.

Causes of Lymphedema

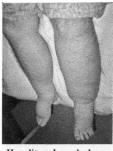

Primary Idiopathic Lymphedema — can be present at birth or develop later in life. It can be either congenital or hereditary. Congenital — present at birth from unknown causes or associated with arterial/

Hereditary Lymphedema

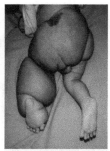

Congenital Lymphedema

23

venous abnormalities as with *Klippel-Trenaunay Syndrome, hemangioma* or *lymphangioma*. Hereditary — only about 10% of primary lymphedema cases are inherited.

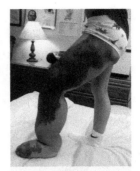

Klippel-Trenaunay

1. Primary Lymphedema Praecox — is the most common form of primary lymphedema appearing during puberty, mostly in girls, and usually affects one lower extremity.

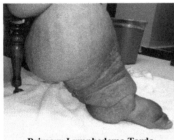

Primary Lymphedema Tarda

2. Primary Lymphedema Tarda — occurs in both males and females. The onset is sudden without any apparent cause and occurs most often between the ages of 35 and 45 years. It can affect one or both extremities, though bilateral (both legs) lymphedema is primarily seen in women.

Secondary or Acquired Lymphedema —develops as a result of:

1. Post surgery — following surgical removal of a cancerous lesion/tumor with lymph node dissection. In most cases, the onset of lymphedema occurs within 24-36 months following surgery. However, it can develop weeks, months, or even years later. It is very important to follow strict guidelines to safeguard against the occurrence of lymphedema.

2. Radiation — can damage otherwise healthy lymph nodes and lymphatic

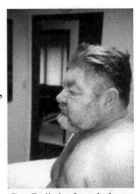

Post-Radiation Lymphedema

vessels, causing scar tissue to form and interrupting the normal flow of lymph fluid. It is important to closely monitor radiated areas for any skin changes, such as inflammation, erythemia (extreme redness) or blistering.

3. During and After Chemotherapy — when it is unwisely administered, such as intravenous instillations into the affected arm or area.

4. Repeated Aspirations of a Seroma — often results in an infection which can trigger lymphedema.

5. Deep Vein Thrombosis — untreated venous insufficiency and varicose veins can create lymphatic/venous imbalance.

6. Infection — when normal lymphatic pathways are interrupted as in an affected lymphedema body part, the protein-rich lymph fluid contained therein begins to stagnate, creating an environment favorable for the growth of bacteria. An infection can occur even though nothing has penetrated the surface of the skin. *Cellulitis* can occur when lymph fluids stagnate under the surface of the skin. The resulting effects are a very red, hot, blistery, swollen, painful, and tender skin intolerant of anything touching it, especially any kind of compression.

Remember: Five symptoms of imminent infection
Red — Hot — Swollen — Hard — Painful

Whenever you experience these signs/symptoms, phone your primary care physician immediately for antibiotic therapy. This kind of infection occurs very quickly, is very painful, and may take several days' convalescence before the infection subsides. (see *Signs of Infection*)

7. Severe Traumatic Injury — severe injury or trauma to a body part in which its lymphatic system is either interrupted or damaged, may trigger the onset of lymphedema.

8. Disease — e.g. *Filariasis* occurs as a result of a bite from an infected mosquito, producing filarial larvae which enter the lymphatic system. When larvae mature into adult worms, they occlude peripheral lymphatic vessels, causing a severe lymphedema known as *Elephantiasis*. There are over 10 million cases in India alone. Peripheral lymphatic vessels are also damaged in the disease *Leprosy*, of which there are 45-50 million cases world-wide.

9. Spontaneous — there is seemingly no reason why lymphedema occurred.

Note: These 3 "happenings" can cause lymphedema:

- surgery + lymph node dissection + radiation = you have a 55-65% chance of developing lymphedema
- surgery alone = you have a 10-15% chance of developing lymphedema
- surgery + lymph node dissection = you have a 25-30% chance of developing lymphedema

— and it can happen at any time.

Signs of Lymphedema

- Persistent swelling in an extremity, usually first noticed in the hands or feet
- A heavy or full sensation in the limb/limbs or affected part
- Skin feeling tight, a heavy or achy feeling
- Decreased flexibility in the joints, especially the knee, elbow, ankle, or wrist
- Swelling that is persistent — it may come and go at first but then it remains
- Difficulty fitting into clothing in a specific area
- Ring, watch, or bracelet feeling tight
- Prickly, burning, or itching sensations in the affected part/area
- Increased swelling in an area that sometimes recedes at night but remains as the body is vertical for a long period of time

After breast surgery with lymph node dissection, the first signs of lymphedema may be a warm, burning, or prickly sensation in the affected axilla (armpit). After surgery some women have lack of sensation on the affected side: chest area, inner upper arm, and axilla. When this occurs, it is very important to visually check for, and be even more aware of, any swelling or changes in these areas. This can be done by visually comparing the affected side with the unaffected side, detecting gradual or sudden tightness of bra bands and straps, garments appearing too small or too tight, especially across the chest and upper arm, and manually feeling for "swollen tissue."

Stages of Lymphedema

Latent Stage — no apparent symptoms

Stage I — (mild) **"pitting"** — when the area is pressed, it indents and holds indentation. Usually the affected area is normal or almost normal in size upon wakening in the AM and is reversible upon elevation.

Stage II — (moderate) **"non pitting"** — affected area has spongy consistency and bounces back without any indentation when pressed.

Stage III — (severe) irreversible — usually the limb is very large and the tissue is hard and fibrotic.

When lymphedema remains untreated, protein-rich fluid continues to accumulate in the tissues, leading to an increase in swelling and a hardening or *fibrosis*. In this state, the swollen area becomes a perfect culture medium for bacteria and subsequent infections, decrease or loss of functioning occurs, the skin begins to break down, chronic infections or *cellulitis* of the area may be frequent, and sometimes irreversible complications occur. In the most severe cases, untreated lymphedema can develop into a rare form of lymphatic cancer known as *lymphangiosarcoma*.

Prevention of Lymphedema

Pre-surgical

♦ If you are predisposed, get informed about lymphedema prior to surgery.
♦ Measure both limbs or pre-surgical area for future reference. Get clear instructions in home care on how to manage any drains that have been inserted during surgery.

- If lymphedema is present or if conditions exist that could cause lymphedema, wear a compression garment on the affected limb/area during any surgical procedure, or have it applied immediately post-surgery.
- In the case of surgery for breast cancer, use an indelible pen and write on the arm of the side of the affected breast: e.g., **Do not touch this arm!**
- Your physician may prescribe an antibiotic prior to any surgical procedure. If you have been diagnosed with lymphedema, this will safeguard against the possibility of infection.

In the Hospital
- Post a large sign on and above your hospital bed stating: **NO blood pressure, NO IVs, NO injections, NO blood drawn.**
- Continue to wear a compression garment on the limb/ area of the surgical side. This will deter any injections or taking of blood pressure.
- If lymphedema is present, wear the compression garment at all times while admitted, except during sleep.
- Upon discharge, wear soft, comfortable, loose-fitting undergarments.
- Wearing TED (anti-emboli) stockings during surgery or having a sequential pump applied post-surgery will assist in lymph return and guard against increased swelling.

In your Doctor's office
- Make all staff members aware: **NO chemotherapy administered in affected arm/limb, NO Blood pressure, and NO Injections.**
- If referred to a physical therapist, seek the help of a certified lymphedema therapist to avoid any complications.

Laboratory testing

♦ Refuse blood draws, IVs, injections, and taking blood pressure on affected limb.

Convalescence

♦ Post surgical drains: watch signs/symptoms of infection, empty drain frequently, keep dressings clean.

Apply good skin care to affected areas. Any break in the skin can open the way for bacteria to enter. It is very important to maintain good healthy skin: keep it clean, soft, and supple, and safeguard against any cuts, bites, or breaks in the surface.

Stay in good health by following good healthy habits, especially good nutrition, sleep habits, good skin care, and daily exercise, keep a positive attitude, and avoid anything that jeopardizes good health.

Maintain an ideal weight with a well-balanced, low-sodium, high-fiber diet. Avoid smoking. No alcoholic beverages. The diet should include protein that is easily digested, such as chicken, fish, and tofu. *Drink plenty of water,* unless otherwise directed by your physician. We suggest 1/2 your weight in ounces of water. For example, if you weigh 150 pounds, we recommend a minimum of 75 ounces/day. Any other fluids ingested are a bonus. Water and fluid intake should be increased gradually giving the body a chance to satisfactorily cleanse the tissues, excrete wastes and maintain your proper body fluid levels.

Life-long steps for prevention

Lymphedema can occur immediately post-operatively, within a few months, a couple of years, or 20 or more years after cancer treatment.

With proper education and care, Lymphedema can be avoided, or if it develops, kept under control.

Follow These Instructions:

- Do not ignore any slight swelling. Consult your physician immediately if you detect any swelling.

- Never allow injections, IVs, blood pressure, or other invasive therapy in the affected arm or area.

- Keep the area "at risk" clean and healthy by applying good skin care including lotions.

- Avoid vigorous, repetitive movements against resistance with the affected limb, e.g., scrubbing, pushing, pulling.

- Avoid heavy lifting or wearing shoulder bags over the affected area.

- Do not wear tight jewelry or bands around affected areas. Including: rings, bracelets, belts, and in the case of breast surgery, check the bra straps and band for pressure points.

- Avoid extreme temperature changes – hot and cold.

- Avoid any type of trauma, e.g., bruises, cuts, animal scratches, bites, sunburn, or burns.

- Wear gloves when doing house and/or garden work to avoid any trauma to the skin or dirt/bacteria invading the tissue.

- Keep nails trimmed but avoid cutting the cuticles unless done by a professional. Purchase your own equipment and supplies to prevent infection through contamination from others' use.

- Exercise is important, but do not overtire an affected area. Everything is done in moderation. Recommended exercises: walking, swimming, light aerobics, cycling, and specifically designed ballet or yoga. Do not lift over 10 pounds. Always wear a well-fitted gradient compression garment during exercise.

- When traveling by air, wear a compression garment and in most instances, reinforce it with compression bandages and/or a higher-grade compression garment. This is the time to increase fluid intake, especially water.

- Wear a well-fitted bra. If a breast form is being worn, make sure it is lightweight and protected in a prosthesis cover.

- When removing hair from the body, use an electric razor instead of a razor blade.

- Wear a well-fitted compression garment during waking hours. At least every 4-6 months check with a lymphedema specialist to see if your garment is compatible with your lymphedema.

Warning!
If a rash, blistering, redness, fever, or increase in temperature in the affected area occurs, consult your physician immediately for antibiotic therapy. These are signs of an impending infection and could mean a worsening of lymphedema.

Prevention
is
Not
a Cure.

If you are a cancer and/or lymphedema patient, it is important that you stay in control of your ongoing cancer and lymphedema checkups and continued maintenance.

Steps to Prevent Upper Extremity Lymphedema
– Who is at Risk?

At risk is anyone who has had either a simple mastectomy, lumpectomy, or modified radical mastectomy in combination with axillary node dissection and, often, radiation therapy. Lymphedema can occur postoperatively either immediately, within a few months, a couple years, or several years after cancer therapy. **With proper education and care, lymphedema can be avoided or, if it develops, kept well under control.**

The following instructions should be reviewed carefully pre-operatively and discussed with your physician or lymphedema specialist:

♦ Absolutely do not ignore any slight increase of swelling In the arm, hand, fingers, neck, or chest wall. *(Consult your physician immediately.)*

♦ Never allow an injection, IV or a blood drawing in the affected arm(s). Wear a lymphedema Alert bracelet. *(Call 1-800-541-3259 for information.)*

♦ Have blood pressure checked on the unaffected arm, or on the leg *(thigh)* if both are affected.

♦ Keep the "at risk" arm spotlessly clean. Use lotion *(Eucerin* or *Lymphoderm)* after bathing. Thoroughly dry — gently — all creases and in-between fingers.

♦ Avoid vigorous, repetitive movements against resistance with the affected arm (e.g., *scrubbing, pushing, pulling).*

34

- Avoid heavy lifting with the affected arm. Never carry heavy handbags or bags with over-the-shoulder straps.

- Do not wear tight jewelry or elastic bands around affected finger, wrist or arm.

- Avoid extreme temperature changes when bathing, washing dishes (no sauna or hot tub). Protect the arm from the sun.

- Avoid any type of trauma *(bruising, cuts, sunburn or other burns, sports injuries, insect bites, cat scratches).*

- Wear gloves while doing housework, gardening, or any type of work that could result in even a minor injury.

- When manicuring your nails, avoid cutting your cuticles. Inform your manicurist to use only sterilized equipment and your own polish.

- Exercise is important, but consult your lymphedema specialist. Do not overtire an arm at risk. If it starts to ache, lie down, elevate it and apply a gradient compression sleeve if you have one. ***Recommended exercises:*** *swimming, water aerobics, cycling, walking, light floor aerobics, and yoga.*

- When traveling by air, patients with lymphedema, or those at risk, should wear a gradient compression sleeve. Additional gradient bandaging or a higher grade compression garment may be necessary on a long flight. Always increase your water intake when traveling.

- Patients with large breasts should wear a lighter breast prosthesis so as not to put too much pressure on the

lymph nodes above the collar bone. Soft padded shoulder straps may be needed to avoid added pressure on the shoulders. Wear a well-fit bra, one that is comfortable and supportive.

♦ Use an electric razor to remove hair, making sure it is maintained properly and has newly-replaced heads.

♦ Patients with lymphedema should wear a well-fitted gradient compression sleeve during all waking hours. At least every 4-6 months, see your lymphedema specialist for follow-up care. If the sleeve is too loose, either the arm has reduced or the sleeve is no longer viable and must be replaced.

♦ *Warning:* If you notice a rash, itching, redness, pain, increase of temperature or fever, consult your physician immediately. These might be signs of an impending infection and could be the beginning or worsening of lymphedema. (see *Signs of Infection*)

♦ Maintain your ideal weight with a well-balanced, low-sodium, high-fiber diet. Avoid smoking and alcohol use. Your diet should contain easily digested protein such as fish, poultry, or tofu.

♦ Lymphedema is a high-protein edema, but eating too little protein will not reduce the protein element in the lymph fluid. Rather, this may weaken the connective tissue and worsen the condition.

Steps to Prevent Lower Extremity Lymphedema
– Who is at Risk?

At risk is anyone who has had gynecological, melanoma, prostate, kidney, bladder or colon cancer in combination with inguinal or abdominal node dissection and, often, radiation therapy. Lymphedema can occur immediately postoperatively, within a few months, a couple years or several years after cancer therapy. **With proper education and care, lymphedema can be avoided or, if it develops, kept well in control.**

The following instructions should be reviewed carefully pre-operatively and discussed with your physician or lymphedema specialist.

♦ Absolutely do not ignore any slight increase of swelling in the toes, foot, ankle, leg, abdomen, or genitals. *(Consult your physician immediately.)*

♦ Never allow an injection, IV or a blood-drawing in the affected leg(s). Wear a lymphedema Alert necklace. *(Call 1-800-541-3259 for information.)*

♦ Keep the "at risk" leg spotlessly clean. Use lotion *(Eucerin* or *Lymphoderm)* after bathing. Thoroughly dry — gently — any creases and between the toes.

♦ Avoid vigorous, repetitive movements against resistance with the affected leg(s).

♦ Do not wear socks, stockings, or undergarments with tight elastic bands.

- Avoid extreme temperature changes when bathing or while washing dishes (no sauna or hot tub). Protect the leg from the sun.

- Avoid any type of trauma *(bruising, cuts, sunburn, or other burns, sports injuries, insect bites, cat scratches).*

- When manicuring your nails, avoid cutting your cuticles. Inform your pedicurist to use only sterilized equipment and your own nail polish.

- Exercise is important, but consult your lymphedema specialist. Do not overtire a leg at risk. If it starts to ache, lie down, elevate it, and apply a gradient compression stocking if you have one. (*Recommended exercises: swimming, water aerobics, cycling, walking, light floor aerobics, and yoga.*)

- When traveling by air, patients with lymphedema, or those at risk, should wear a gradient compression stocking. Additional gradient bandaging may be necessary on a long flight. Always increase your water intake when traveling.

- Use an electric razor to remove hair, making sure it is maintained properly and has newly-replaced heads.

- Patients with lymphedema should wear a well-fit gradient compression stocking during all waking hours. At least every 4-6 months, see your lymphedema specialist for follow-up care. If the stocking is too loose, either the leg has reduced or the stocking is no longer viable and must be replaced.

- *Warning:* If you notice a rash, itching, redness, pain increase of temperature or fever, consult your physician immediately. These might be signs of an impending infection and could be the beginning or worsening of lymphedema. (see *Signs of infection*)

♦ Maintain your ideal weight with a well-balanced, low-sodium, high-fiber diet. Avoid smoking and alcohol use. Your diet should contain easily digested protein such as fish, poultry, or tofu.

♦ Lymphedema is a high-protein edema, but eating too little protein will not reduce the protein element in the lymph fluid. Rather, this may weaken the connective tissue and worsen the condition.

♦ Always wear closed-toe shoes (high tops or well-fitted boots) - n*o sandals, slippers, or going barefoot.*

♦ See a podiatrist once a year to check and treat for fungus, ingrown toenails, calluses, pressure areas, athlete's foot.

♦ Wear clean socks and hosiery at all times.

♦ Use baby powder on feet, especially if you perspire a great deal. Be sure to wear rubber gloves when pulling on stockings. Talcum powder behind the knee often helps to prevent rubbing and irritation.

Recommendations for Patients With Lymphedema

◆ Always try to use a positive-reinforcement system of rewards.

◆ Change limb position often rather than let it rest in one position too long.

◆ Try to sleep so that your body weight is not pressing on the limb (slows circulation). If at all possible, sleep with arm elevated above heart level, as the lymph pathways from the arm area will be more direct.

◆ Exercise is good for shorter rather than longer periods so as not to over-tire the limb. Always wear a gradient compression garment when exercising.

◆ Carry bags and heavy loads on the unaffected side.

◆ Use the unaffected limb for blood pressure measurements, injections; avoid all injury to the limb (e.g., shaving a limb should be done carefully with an electric razor).

◆ Have any infections and unusual redness (inflammation) attended to immediately by a medical doctor. (see *Signs of Infection*)

◆ Have MLD performed immediately on recent hematoma/bruising, making sure first there are no venous problems such as blood clots.

◆ Keep the limb out of the sun as much as possible and especially avoid sunburns.

◆ Clothing should be loose and comfortable with no tight constriction on the affected side (e.g. bra straps, elasticized socks or under garments).

- Wear a wristwatch only on the unaffected side, as it may trap bacteria or pinch the skin on the affected side. Tight jewelry may have the same effect.

- Keep the affected limb as clean and supple as possible by using cleansing lotions and/or mild soaps.

- When taking a shower or bath, use tepid-warm (rather than hot) temperatures, as heat will make the swelling worse.

- Wash bandages and DFG (directional flow garment) once a week and compression garments daily, according to the manufacturer's instructions, and air-dry away from direct sunlight.

- Report to your lymphedema therapist any chaffing, redness, indentation, looseness or tightness of the compression garment.

- If a prosthesis is used, wear a light one on the affected side.

- Keep your weight down as much as possible and try to lose weight if you are overweight.

- A well-balanced, low-salt, high-fiber diet is recomended. Avoid smoking and alcohol use. Lymphedema is a high protein edema, but eating too little protein will not reduce the protein element in the lymph fluid. Rather, this may weaken the connective tissue and worsen the condition. Diet should contain easily-digested protein, e.g., chicken, fish, tofu.

- Diuretics, which increase fluid elimination, are no longer favored in the treatment of lymphedema, because they can exacerbate protein build-up in the tissues.

- Special precautions, such as wearing protective gloves or footwear, may be necessary to avoid injuring the affected region.

Signs and Symptoms of Impending Infection

Lymphedema infections manifest themselves in many different ways and are individual to each patient.

5 Main Symptoms:
Red — Hot — Swollen — Hard — Painful

- Malaise (feeling lethargic)
- Rash or itchy sensation
- Redness and/or red streaks on affected parts
- Increase in body temperature, fever
- Sudden increase in girth of affected area
- Affected area becomes very swollen, hard and "hot" to touch
- Onset of pain and/or severe discomfort in the affected area
- Achy or heavy feeling in joints of an affected limb with pain upon movement.
- If any of these occur, consult your Primary Care Physician immediately for antibiotic therapy.

Note: Any generalized infection such as the flu may affect a lymphedematous body part. Patients have reported changes in an affected area during generalized illness. It is important to take special care to prevent infection from occurring in the affected lymphedematous body part.

During Acute Phase of Infection:

♦ **Do Not** apply compression – it will cause pain and move infection into other parts of the body.

♦ Skin Care
   - wash affected area several times per day.
   - dry thoroughly and apply water-base antibacterial
     lotion.

♦ 48-72 hours after onset of antibiotic therapy: Combined Decongestive Therapy (CDT) must begin to decongest and reduce affected area. If the infection is treated with antibiotics at the very onset of symptoms, gradient compression may be applied within 48-72 hours, **if gradient compression does not cause pain.**

♦ If gradient compression causes pain, wait 12 more hours and attempt to re-apply compression.

♦ Limit activities, and rest as much as possible to allow the body to fight the infection.

♦ Eat a well-balanced, nutritious diet, preferably small, frequent servings, as tolerated.

- Drink plenty of fluids, especially water, to flush out impurities from the tissues. The optimum is 1/2 your weight in ounces of water, daily.

Compresses for Treating Infection During Acute Phase

Over the years of our treating *cellulitis* associated with lymphedema, we have found that vinegar compresses, applied to an acute cutaneous (skin) infection, work very well.

Rationale: The skin has an acidic 5.5ph. Vinegar is also acidic. but has a slightly different ph. Bacteria which cause infection thrive in a certain ph. By changing the ph of the skin slightly, these bacteria cannot survive. In addition, the pores of the skin absorb anything applied to the skin's surface. Vinegar solution penetrates the pores of the skin into the underlying tissues, killing bacteria. This relieves tissue sensitivity exteriorly, the antibiotics kill the bacteria interiorly.

Application Directions:
1. Mix equal parts white vinegar & water.
2. Put down a sheet of plastic to protect furniture.
3. Apply towel around affected area.
4. Using a basting syringe, wet towel with vinegar/water solution. Reapply as towel dries.
5. As the skin becomes less sensitive, full-strength vinegar solution may be applied. If it burns, dilute vinegar with water.
6. Continue to apply compresses until skin sensitivity and redness have subsided.

Lymphedema Care Kit

**When traveling, always carry your
"Lymphedema Care Kit." This should include:**

- Small bar of soap & washcloth
- *Alps* lotion
- *Lymphoderm* lotion
- A&D ointment
- Antibiotic ointment
- Stockinette - tubular gauze
- Finger/toe bandages
- Skin adhesive
- Roll of tape
- Short stretch and/or long stretch bandage rolls
- "Swell spots"- pressure pads for isolated problem areas
- Rubber gloves
- Artiflex padding or foam
- Directional Flow Garment
- Compression garments
- Garment donning aid, e.g., Slip-eze
- Oral antibiotics
- *Lymphedema Self-Care Manual*

Lymphedema is very unpredictable. When environmental conditions change, lymphedema changes, too. Knowing how to care for yourself, and having the required supplies and equipment at hand, gives you the power to be prepared for whatever you do — wherever you are.

Conditions That May Complicate Or Worsen Lymphedema

- Radiation
- Extreme heat
- Chemotherapy
- Reconstructive surgery
- Any invasive treatment/surgery
- Any surgery in the affected quadrant
- Infections
- Air travel
- Blood pressure on affected arm
- Increased altitudes - above 4,000 ft.
- Breast Implant preparation
- Repeated aspirations of body fluids
- Injections on the affected arm or leg
- Body massage of the affected quadrant
- Liposuction of the affected area

The butterfly is the
international symbol for
Lymphedema.

Chapter 2

Lymphedema Treatment

Combined Decongestive Therapy (CDT)

Staffed by medically-educated, Certified Lymphedema Therapists, a professional lymphedema treatment center offers a program that effectively treats the special needs of those afflicted with lymphedema. In the case of breast cancer, particular emphasis is on early treatment post-breast surgery to reduce pain and relieve edema/swelling. Specific treatment includes attention to:

- cervical lymph nodes
- scar or incision
- affected arm and movement therapy of the shoulder joint
- skin area receiving radiation therapy

The recommended treatment for lymphedema consists of an all-inclusive therapy known as **Combined Decongestive Therapy (CDT)** which includes: manual lymph drainage, gradient bandaging, remedial exercises, circumferential measurements of affected limb, instructions in diet and nutrition, skin care, measure and fitting gradient compression garments, and a home maintenance program designed for the patient's involvement in his/her therapy. The length of the intensive phase of CDT is dependent upon the severity of the lymphedema case, patient's age, amount of time the patient has (work schedule, etc.), if the patient needs assistance with care (ability to perform self-care), the financial situation, and insurance coverage.

Goal of CDT is to decongest congested tissues, thereby bringing about reduction of the affected part.
After an initial medical examination and development of an individual treatment plan (protocol for therapy), CDT commences. Each therapy session decongests the involved quadrant of the body starting with the trunk, advancing to the swollen extremity, always moving fluids from distal (farthest part) to proximal (nearest).

The Steps to Achieve CDT:

1. **Circumferential Measurements of Affected Limb/ limbs** — Measurements around the limb are taken every 4 cm up the limb and recorded in mm, liters, and pounds. This serves as a baseline to measure reduction of fluid volume. As each session of intensive CDT progresses, the area is measured at the same 4 cm locations on the limb. When the affected area is the same, or nearly the same volume or circumferential measurements for 3 consecutive days, and there exists no further fibrosis or infection, the area is fit with a gradient compression garment to maintain reduction.

2. **Manual Lymph Drainage (MLD)** — This empties and decompresses obstructed lymphatic vessels. (see *Chapter 3)*

3. **Proper Skin Care** — The affected area is cleansed, rinsed thoroughly and lotions applied. Since padding and gradient bandages are applied for an extended amount of time, the skin must be moisturized and protected before each re-bandaging. A water-base lotion is applied first, followed by a heavier cream or ointment. This serves as a barrier to hold moisture in, and protects the skin from long term bandage pressure, especially at the creases, joints, and folds.

4. Gradient Compression Bandaging — Following skin care, the affected area is protected with a loosely woven cotton tubular wrap. Soft cotton padding or foam is then applied, followed by pressure bandages that are applied gradiently. Short stretch bandages are used to move fluids while the patient is exercising or moving. Unlike Ace bandages which move fluids while a patient is resting, eg., ankle sprain, short stretch bandages move fluids while a patient is moving. Thus, gradient compression bandaging:

- moves fluids out of congested areas into healthy adjacent lymphatic channels
- decongests or breaks-up fibrotic areas
- reduces the size and volume of the affected area
- prevents the re-accumulation of fluids.

5. Gradient Compression Garments — Specific to the area, these garments can be either "ready-to-wear" or "custom made." Gradient compression garments maintain fluid reduction of the affected area once CDT is completed. (see *Chapter 4*)

6. Diet and Nutrition — With weight gain, fat cells become larger, and fluid movement through affected tissues is impeded. This can be compared to water flowing over boulders rather than over smooth cement. When weight loss occurs, there is also a corresponding loss of girth and weight in the affected are as well as in the unaffected area. (see *Chapter 10*)

7. Remedial Exercises — During intensive CDT and following the initial bandaging phase, instructions for exercises specific for each lymphedema condition and affected body part are given. While gradient compression bandages are in place, exercises are performed to move fluids more effectively. (see *Chapter 6*)

8. Instructions in Self-Care — Education in self-care is given as CDT progresses. This includes every phase of CDT and is patient specific. When intensive therapy is completed, the patient is fit in a gradient compression garment and placed on a home-maintenance program designed to prevent recurrence.

9. Gradient Sequential Pump
Patient needs met:
- Easily applied
- Home self-treatment care
- Daily usage
- Volume reduction
- Fibrosis prevention
- Tissue softening

10. Continued Prophylactic Methods (Maintenance) — While in most cases lymphedema is not curable, proper treatment and maintenance can reduce the size of the affected body part and restore the patient to a full and productive lifestyle. Though lymphedema patients and their care givers would like the affected part to return to "normal" size, good maintenance may be soft tissue, no thickening or fibrosis, and absence of infection. Good maintenance of lymphedema requires regular manual lymph drainage (MLD) treatments and wearing an up-to -date gradient compression garment.

Phases of Combined Decongestive Therapy (CDT)

Phase I — **Intensive Phase**
The goal is to decongest and reduce large fluid volumes and break up fibrosis. Fifteen to twenty (15-20) consecutive treatments are scheduled for 3-4 weeks until circumferential measurements of the affected area/limb are the same or nearly the same for 3 consecutive days. The patient is measured for a gradient compression garment and must continue with bandage compression until garment arrives or is fit. (see *Page 58)*

Phase II — **Transitional Phase**
The goal is to "teach the body" to continue to move fluids into collateral pathways. Even though this phase may last up to six months, some patients continue it for an extended period of time to prevent any complications and to increase reduction of fluids. A gradient compression garment is worn during the day, and bandaging over a directional flow garment is done at night. (see *Page 64)*

Phase III — **Maintenance Phase**
(Living with Lymphedema)
Schedule manual lymph drainage (MLD) at regular intervals with a qualified lymphedema therapist who will monitor the lymphedema condition and educate the patient about new techniques and supplies needed for management of lymphedema. Patients wear gradient compression garments daily. Garment is to be applied when awakening in the AM and removed before bedtime. (see *Page 87)*

Goals of Combined Decongestive Therapy (CDT)

1. Decrease lymph volume — When tissues are decongested through compression, fluids and wastes move out of the affected area, bringing about reduction in lymph volume.

2. Improve shape of affected area — Reduction of lymph volume gives better shape to an affected body part.

3. Improve condition of the skin — Skin of the affected area is unhealthy and dry due to stagnation of wastes in underlying tissues. Reduction in lymph volume also means reduction in body wastes, therefore, healthier skin.

4. Decrease and/or effectively eliminate fibrosis — Using gradient compression bandaging on top of padding results in breaking up fibrous connective tissues.

5. Reduce pain — CDT reduces swollen body parts that are uncomfortable and heavy.

6. Increase mobility and increase range of motion — Excess lymph fluids in an affected limb can settle in and around the joints inhibiting movement. Once fluid reduction begins in the tissues through CDT, the joints are also relieved of stagnant fluids.

7. Increase efficiency of the immune system — The lymphatic system is part of the immune system, since its chief purpose is to carry out wastes and fight infection. When body wastes are removed through CDT, the lymphatic system works more efficiently.

8. Work Concurrently with Antibiotic Therapy – To reduce infection. Compression begins 48-72 hours after initial dose of antibiotic therapy.

9. Empower the patient — Teaching the principles of a home care regimen specific to each patient is very important for self-care and maintenance.

10. Enhance Quality of life — The health of our body directly affects how we feel and how we live.

Effects of Combined Decongestive Therapy (CDT)

- Reduces pain
- Relaxes smooth muscle
- Increases lymph drainage
- Reduces swelling and fibrosis
- Increases efficiency of immune system
- Decongests affected lymphedematous areas
- Increases mobility and range of motion
- Assists in reducing inflammatory and infectious processes during concurrent antibiotic therapy

Protocol for Home Care During Intensive Phase of Combined Decongestive Therapy (CDT)

Intensive Phase

Each Day of Treatment — (*performed under strict guidance and supervision of a Lymphedema Specialist*):

♦ After awakening and using the restroom, begin exercises with bandages on. Do each exercise 15 times, 2-3x/day.

♦ Always remember to inhale while at rest and exhale while exercising.

♦ Remove bandages and bathe. Apply special skin care on the affected area using cleansing products prescribed. Rinse well and allow to dry thoroughly. Apply cream/lotion/ointment to affected areas as instructed.

Finger & Toe Bandaging — (*Before attempting this, get proper instructions from a Lymphedema Specialist*):

Apply stockinette from tip of toes or fingertips up the entire limb. Then fold back stockinette to ankle or wrist. For the hand, cut a small opening in the stockinette for the thumb. Using appropriate width, soft elastic cotton roll (*Elastamul*), secure the roll at the wrist, wrapping one time around. For the foot, secure the roll at the ball of the foot. Using a "figure of 8" technique, roll across the top of the hand (or foot) toward the finger (or toe), then wrap the finger (or toe) 3 times around securely, but not tight. Roll the bandage away from the finger (or toe) over the top of the hand (or foot), down the other side of the wrist (or foot) from which you brought it up. (Always remember when wrapping the hand or foot, the bandage is rolled out across the top of the hand or foot "up one side and down the other" – in a figure of 8 technique). Continue doing this with each finger or toe until all fingers or toes are covered. If there is bandage left, continue wrapping up the arm or foot until the entire roll is used. Do not cut bandages.

Webbing – using 1" *Elastamul*, secure it at the wrist or ball of the foot as you did above. Using the same "figure of 8" technique, go around each finger or toe one time at the base securely but not tight. When all have been webbed, continue wrapping the bandage up the hand or foot until the entire roll is used. Do not cut bandages.

Pull the stockinette down over the bandages. For the fingers, cut a thumb hole and slide the thumb through the stockinette opening.

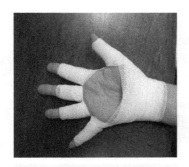
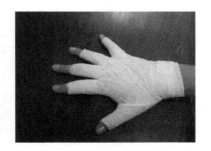

Palm up, open hand   Palm down, open hand

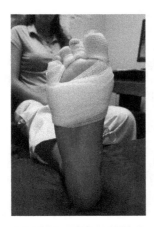
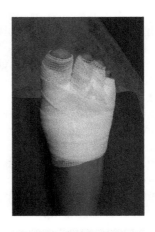

Sole of foot   Top of foot

Bandaging the Arm or Leg:

Apply cotton stockinette over affected limb, making sure to eliminate any creases. Next, pad the hand or foot with appropriate padding designed for that part. Then, using roll padding, continue to wrap the limb from farthest to nearest part of the limb (distal to proximal), overlapping each roll about 1/3 as you progress up the limb. Second, third and fourth rolls of padding may be needed to complete the wrap, depending upon the length of the limb and the desired depth of padding necessary to bring about decongestion of the tissues. The padding is to be wrapped snug.

Next, apply short stretch roll bandages using the 6cm first on the hand or 8cm first on the foot, as instructed. Begin at the base of the fingers or toes and wrap around 3 times in one place, being sure that the fingers and toes are spread while wrapping. Then follow with a "figure of 8" wrap technique around the wrist or ankle showing 1/4" to 1/2" of the previous bandage as you wrap up the hand or foot to the wrist or ankle. Good coverage will feel almost like a cast. Be sure to cover the palm of the hand around the thumb, and for the foot, cover the heel adequately. The first bandage will most likely end around the wrist or ankle. Start the second bandage 8cm for the arm or 10cm for the leg where the first bandage ended, overlapping the bandage, showing 1/3 of the width of the roll. Third, fourth, or fifth bandage rolls may be necessary to completely cover the limb, depending upon the circumference and length of the affected limb. Check for gradient pressure, with the most pressure at the hand/wrist or foot/ankle and decreasing as it goes up the limb. Apply additional bandages where you feel weaknesses, usually around or near the wrist or ankle and continue up the limb. As each bandage roll is applied over the previous bandage:

This is the wrapping sequence:
- 1st bandage, show 1/3 of its width;
- 2nd bandage, show 1/2 of its width;
- 3rd bandage and any bandage applied thereafter, show 1/2 of the width.

Always begin each bandage at the wrist or ankle for gradiency. Secure the last bandage with tape and apply stockinette over entire limb over bandages to prevent bandages from telescoping downward and prevent soiling.

Every day you must launder bandages that touch the skin, e.g., stockinette and finger bandages. Short stretch bandage rolls and padding need not be laundered but once a week, except when they are soiled. Wash in a mild soap, like *Dreft* or *Ivory*, in a nylon mesh bag in your washing machine and dry them on low heat or air cycle of your dryer. Then roll them for next day's use. It is necessary to have 2 sets of bandages, one being worn while the other set is being laundered.

If you feel tightness after bandaging, especially around the joint area (elbow or knee) or near the toes or fingers and it becomes unbearable, remove one bandage at a time until it becomes more comfortable. If the bandages remain uncomfortable, remove all bandage rolls, leaving padding, and rewrap. The most important thing is that there is gradient pressure (most pressure at the farthest point of the limb gradually decreasing up the limb – distal to proximal).

From time to time, check the temperature and color of the toes and fingers – nail beds and skin. If they feel cool or appear blue, the bandages may be too tight. It is important to note that an older person may not tolerate tighter bandages as well as a younger person.
In order to achieve maximum lymphedema reduction

during CDT, it is necessary to leave bandages on affected limb/limbs 23/7 (hours/day), only free of bandages long enough to bathe, do skin care, and perform MLD. **Skin care should be done before clean bandages are re-applied.** It is important to rewrap the limb and do skin care A.M. and P.M. to sustain maximum compression. Never apply soiled or used bandages over an affected limb – there is always a higher chance of infection with lymphedema or any edema.

Criteria for Intensive Phase of CDT
(23-hour gradient bandaging)

- **if affected limb is 2-3cm larger circumferentially than the unaffected limb**

- **if fibrosis exists in affected area/limb**

Instructions for Daily Care Following CDT

Transitional Phase

(30–60 days immediately after intensive phase)

Morning:

♦ Before removing directional flow garment (DFG), do the lymphedema exercises as instructed.

♦ While wearing DFG, perform manual lymph drainage on "exits" as detailed on patient specific "protocol for therapy diagram."

♦ Remove DFG and bandages, then bathe as usual.

♦ Apply *Lymphoderm* Lotion, A&D Ointment on very dry areas and creases/folds.

♦ Apply *A lps* Lotion as directed: arm to elbow; leg to knee.

♦ Apply gradient compression garments (stockings, sleeves, gloves, etc.) with the aid of rubber gloves.

♦ Try to wear the gradient compression garments throughout the day.

♦ Rotate your garments according to your needs or as indicated by the condition of your lymphedema.

Evening:

♦ Before removing garment, perform Manual Lymph Drainage on "exits" as protocol is instructed.

♦ Remove gradient compression garments and wash daily.

♦ Wash/cleanse affected limb/area with soap and water, rinse well.

♦ Apply *Lymphoderm* Lotion and A&D Ointment as

directed – *Lymphoderm* Lotion all over and A&D
Ointment in dry or pressure areas.
♦ Bandage toes or fingers if there is residual swelling
from the day.
♦ Apply stockinette if necessary for easier application of
DFG.
♦ Apply DFG garment, to be worn all night. If more
compression is needed due to residual swelling, apply
bandages over the DFG garment and leave on all night.
During the night if there is discomfort, remove
bandages and leave on DFG. (see *Leg Bandaging, page
48*)
♦ Do lymphedema exercises with DFG on.
♦ DFG should be laundered once/week. (see *Chapter 7*)

Diuretics

Diuretics, which increase fluid elimination, are no longer
favored in the treatment of lymphedema, because they can
exacerbate protein build-up in the tissues. At the onset of
their use, diuretics seem to help in removing some excess
fluids from affected areas. Since diuretics remove only
fluids from the body, they cannot remove larger protein
particles that only the lymphatics can transport. These
remaining protein particles left in the tissues continue to
attract and hold body fluids, resulting in continued swelling.

Any time there is swelling, there exists an accumulation of
body wastes in body fluids, and the body does not like
having its own wastes stagnating its tissues. Body fluids
must be in constant motion, or the resulting effects can be
devastating: *fibrosis* (hardened tissues).

For example, if fibrosis exists in an upper arm or leg, fluids
cannot get past this blockage. Swelling will increase in the

lower part of the limb each day fibrosis is not treated. Also, fibrotic areas become more difficult to decongest each day the condition exists.

In addition, increased swelling in the joints leads to fibrosis of joint tissues, bringing about less and less mobility. The longer this condition is left untreated, immobility becomes a grave issue — a cycle whereby the degree of immobility increases with untreated fibrosis.

Chapter 3

Manual Lymph Drainage (MLD)

Developed in Austria in the mid-1930s by Emil and Estrid
Vodder, Mannual Lymph Drainage (MLD) facilitates
removal of wastes, excess water, toxins, bacteria, large
protein molecules and foreign substances from the tissues.
MLD is not a massage. Rather, it is a progressive
technique of lymphatic decompression. It is a slow,
repetitive, rhythmic movement of the hands, using very
light strokes, (approximately 30 mmHg pressure), moving
skin to bring about a gentle pumping action in the tissues.
This pumping action stimulates the weakened lymphatic
system by pushing stagnant lymph fluid through vessels,
allowing the larger venous system to reabsorb the fluid,
thus supporting the development of new collateral channels
through which the lymph can begin to flow. Lymph is
shunted into accessory pathways, bypassing the normal
route of flow. Only highly skilled therapists know how this
is to be accomplished for each individual case. The end
result of MLD is: the removal of excess fluids, soothing
nerves, alleviating pain, having a physiological calming
effect, and supporting immunity.

Manual lymph drainage is performed by certified MLD
therapists who have been specially educated in lymphatic
anatomy, physiology, and pathophysiology. While MLD is
specific for the treatment of lymphedema, it has also been
indicated in the treatment of a number of other conditions,
for example, sprains, dislocations, fractures, burns,
tendonitis, tennis elbow, migraines, headaches, acne,
glaucoma, sinusitis, allergies, pre-and post-cosmetic
surgery, oral and general surgery, carpel tunnel syndrome,
as a decongestant, to minimize scar formation (keloids), and

for acute and chronic edema associated with heart disease and venous insufficiency. MLD can also promote growth and recovery, restore strength, and create a feeling of well being.

Manual lymph drainage is contraindicated —when there is active, not yet treated malignancy, acute inflammation or infection present, a blood clot or thrombosis, and heart related edema.

Mannual Lymph Drainage is used cautiously with these conditions — treated malignancy, chronic inflammation, stabilized thrombosis, low blood pressure, hyperactive thyroid, asthma, tuberculosis, nevus (moles), menstruation, and pregnancy.

Manual lymph drainage is effective for all kinds of lymphedema, including various primary and secondary forms. The sooner the patient receives MLD therapy after the onset of swelling or edema, the quicker the response and the fewer treatments needed.

The effects of MLD are greatest 24–36 hours after therapy. This is when fluids move more efficiently; therefore, it is important to apply gradient compression immediately post treatment.

Criteria Supporting the Action of Mannual Lymph Drainage (MLD)

♦ The treatment room is kept at a comfortable temperature – covering those body parts that are not being treated.
♦ The patient is placed in a comfortable position. This can be difficult when the patient has heavy edematous limbs.
♦ Light and sounds are kept to a minimum so as not to disturb the patient, which would counteract the goal of the treatment.
♦ The therapist's hands need to be warm – cold hands cannot promote lymph drainage.
♦ MLD must *not* be painful. Pain increases the sympathetic tonus causing increased edema and spasm in the draining lymph vessels.
♦ The force of the hand movements must feel pleasant. The strength of pressure depends on the tissue being treated and the patient's sensitivity.
♦ Generally MLD must *not* cause reddening of the skin – this appears when pressure is too heavy.
♦ No lubricants are used except when treatment is performed in areas of the body covered with thick hair.
♦ After MLD treatment there is *a period of rest*, usually 5 –10 minutes. MLD can then continue to have an effect, and blood pressure can return to normal.
♦ The treatment of each illness follows the so-called *Therapy Strokes* where the sequence of movements is matched to the particular symptoms and often combined with movements of affected joints.

Precautions

When the lymphatic system has been impaired, special pre-cautions are necessary to avoid aggravating affected body parts. For example, under no circumstances should blood samples and blood pressure be taken or injections received in an edematous limb or affected quadrant. This would in-crease the possibility of infection and put the patient at con-siderable health risk. In addition, if a compression pump is used aggressively at the onset of lymphedema without prior opening of the fluid channels with manual lymph drainage, the pump could cause further lymph vessel blockage. Gra-dient sequential pneumatic pumps are used in conjunction with a patient-specific directional flow garment (DFG), ap-plied under the pump sleeve. (see *Chapter 9*)

Protocol
for
Therapy

71

Upper Left Quadrant Affected

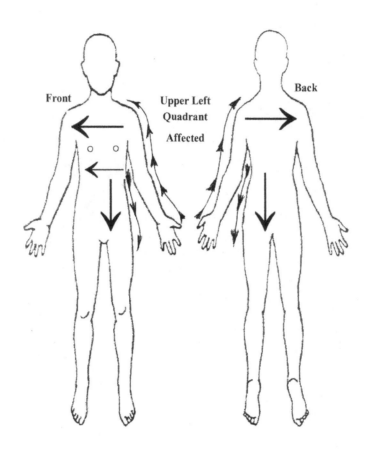

Upper Right Quadrant Affected

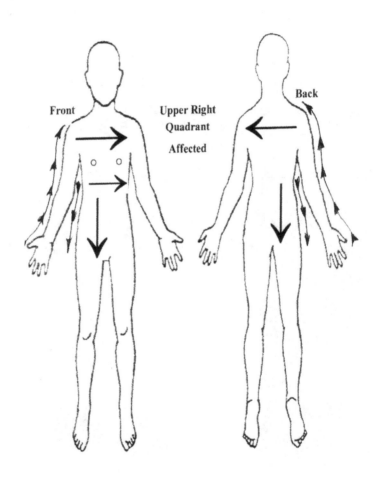

Front

Upper Right
Quadrant

Affected

Back

Upper Bilaterally Affected

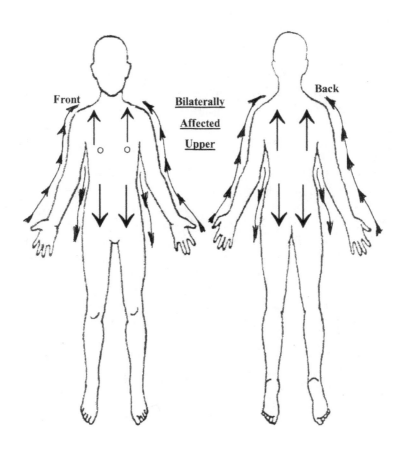

Front

Bilaterally
Affected
Upper

Back

Lower Right Quadrant Affected

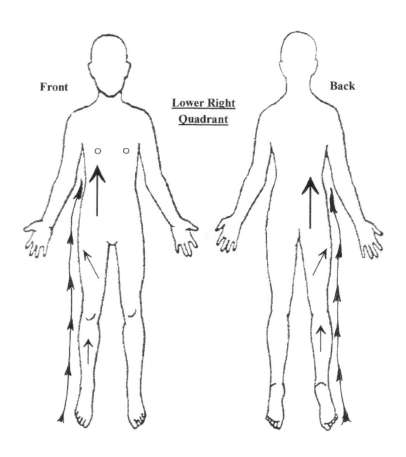

Front

Back

Lower Right
Quadrant

75

Lower Left Quadrant Affected

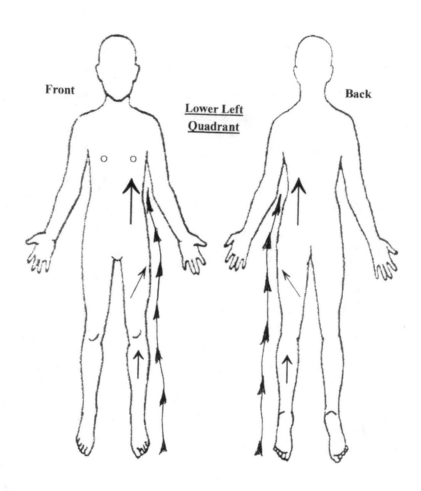

Front

Back

Lower Left
Quadrant

Lower Bilaterally Affected

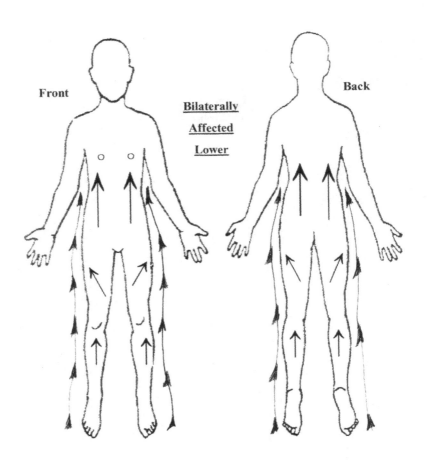

Front

Bilaterally
Affected
Lower

Back

Self Manual Lymph Drainage (Self MLD)

The lymphedema specialist sets protocol for therapy after initial evaluation of each patient. From this, a protocol for home self-care is set and follows the protocol for treatment performed at the lymphedema clinic. A diagram is made detailing a numbering sequence for moving fluids, and the patient and/or home caregivers are instructed in Self Manual Lymph Drainage (Self MLD), basic anatomy and physiology of the lymphatic system, gradient bandaging using padding and short-stretch bandages, and skin care. If wounds are to be dressed, the patient and caregivers are instructed in wound care before applying bandages, gradient compression garments or directional flow garments (DFG).

For instance, in the case of a patient with lymphedema of the right upper quadrant (arm and torso, front and back), fluids are moved across the body, right to left into the left armpit (axilla). Fluids are also moved down across the waist from the right upper torso into the right groin, front and back.

Chapter 4

Gradient Compression Garments

Gradient compression garments ensure that counter pressure is greatest at the most distant part of the limb with gradual decreasing pressure toward the nearest part of the affected area or body. These garments assist the body's natural mechanism for venous and lymph return from the extremity.

According to a report given at the September 1998, National Lymphedema Network Conference held in San Francisco, the percentage ratio of lymphedema fluid reduction compared with garment and exercise compliance time is:

Compliance time	% of reduction
100%	79.0%
50%	39.6%
0-25%	less than 30.0%

Any gradient compression garment over 20 millimeters of mercury pressure (20mmHg) is designated a "medical compression garment" and requires an order from a medical doctor for fitting. Garments can be purchased over the counter as "ready made," if measurements of the affected area adapt to a standard size range. When the affected area is over sized or not within the standard size range, a custom garment is ordered, made to specific limb/area measurements, usually requiring 3-4 weeks delivery. Despite "old ideas," garments are becoming "more fashionable." Colors such as mocha, champagne, barely black, pearl, mink, navy, silky beige, and the "old stand-by" black or white, make wearing compression the *in-Thing* now.

Fabrics are much lighter weight and more sheer, and not like the garments grandmother wore.; skin can actually be seen through the garment. More styles are also available to suit all sizes and compression needs. Ready-made stockings are available in open- or closed-toe styles, to the knee, to the groin, or in pantyhose. Custom garments are made according to the patient's needs as outlined by the lymphedema specialist or the patient's physician. Custom gradient compression garments can be designed for the whole body, e.g., stockings, sleeves, pants, bras, gloves, vests, body suits, socks, booties, and variations thereof, according to each patient's needs.

Despite all the advancements in fabrics, colors, and styles, the difficulty in applying stockings is getting them over the heel. The secret in pulling up any gradient compression garment is patience, a pair of rubber gloves, good skin care, and donning aids such as *A lps* Silicon Lotion, and other useful tools. A qualified lymphedema specialist will give instructions in application of gradient compression garments and skin care during the fitting. Pre-schedule these fittings with your lymphedema specialist to allow sufficient time for necessary measurements and instructions.

Gradient Compression Garments are used for:
- Varicose veins
- Chronic venous insufficiency
- Varicosities associated with pregnancy
- Post-facial surgery
- Burns
- Arm lymphedema following breast surgery
- Post-abdominal surgery
- Venous ulcers
- Post liposuction or sclerotherapy
- Inflammation or swelling during or post radiation

- Vein ligation and stripping
- Any "frequent flyer" who is airborne longer than two hours
- Anyone having a profession/career that calls for standing or sitting for long periods of time

Most of us will experience some form of venous disease in our lifetime. Venous disease can range from a milder form such as superficial varicosities, to severe unsightly leg ulcers. The majority of "leg complaints" are directly related to venous dysfunction.

Accessories — People who wear gradient compression garments, especially thigh high stockings and arm sleeves, often have problems with the garment slipping down. A silicon band at the top of the stocking or sleeve will most generally help to avoid this problem. If a silicon band is applied to any garment, there is an added cost In addition, there are hypoallergenic skin adhesives available which, when they are applied to the skin at the level of the band on the garment, also prevent the garment from creeping down. Even though these skin adhesives are "hypo-allergenic." it is important to do a skin test prior to full application in order to avoid any skin reactions. *Avoid* applying any adhesive on the skin near the axilla (armpit) and/or inguinal (groin). These areas tend to be more sensitive.

Different fabrics in garments bring about different pressure effects, even though they may have the same compression class. For instance, a **circular knit** fabric garment is tapered, shaped cylindrical and has no seams. Once fit on the body part, it conforms to the shape of the body. With creases and folds of the body such as the elbow crease or the back of the knee, circular knit garments can produce a "rubber band" effect and may become uncomfortable over a period of time. Good skin care, making sure the weave of the garment is evenly distributed, can alleviate this, in most instances. If skin irritation persists, consult your lymphedema specialist; a different garment may be necessary. Usually custom-made gradient compression garments are fabricated from **flat knit** fabric. These garments have seams and are made to the shape and size of the body part. Because of the nature of the flat fabric weave, these garments usually move fluids more effectively and, since they are made to specific body measurements, are usually more comfortable.

Care of Gradient Compression Garments — Launder garments daily in tepid water, using a mild soap such as *Dreft or Ivory*, **No Woolite**, rinse well, roll in a fluffy towel to remove any excess water, and hang to dry away from direct heat and sunlight. Also, garments can be placed in a mesh bag and machine washed on delicate cycle using tepid water and a mild soap. Hang to dry as above. Daily laundering not only removes bodily residue, which breaks down elastic fibers, but also laundering returns the garment to its former elasticity. We suggest two (2) garments; one being worn while the second one is being laundered. This extends the life of both garments.

Life of a Garment —- When one garment is worn daily, its life is about 3-4 months. Elastic fibers break down over time and the garment shows signs of "pilling" and rolling down, causing a tourniquet effect. Also the fabric looses its "short stretch" capability, has a sagging effect, and no longer controls swelling. The affected body part begins to swell as tissues retain more fluids and bodily wastes, increasing the chance of infection.

Alternately wearing two garments gives the patient more flexibility and also increases both garments' lives to 6+ months. **It is very important to keep garments current in**

order to control swelling.

Never stand or sit too long while wearing any gradient support stockings. A 90-degree bend or lack of movement will cause pooling of fluids below the bend. Exercise or muscular movement moves fluids more efficiently. Gradient compression garments are not worn at night during sleep because we never sleep with our legs or arms continuously straight out; we sleep with our knees and elbows bent. Gradient compression garments are designed to move fluids from the lower arm/leg, with most pressure at the wrist/ankle, up the arm/leg, and the pressure decreases as fluids move into the upper limb. These garments move fluids while the patient is in motion. Depending upon the mmHg pressure in the garment, compression differences in gradient compression garments bring about changes in pressure at specific points on the limb. The following graph illustrates, for instance, how pressure decreases up the leg as compression in stockings increases at the ankle when pantyhose are worn.

How gradient compression works:

Point on Leg/Arm	15-20mmHg	20-30mmHg (CC-1)	30-40mmHg (CC-2)
Ankle/wrist 100%	18.0mmHg	26.0mmHg	36.0mmHg
Knee/elbow 70%	12.6mmHg	18.2mmHg	25.2mmHg
Groin/armpit 40%	7.2mmHg	10.4mmHg	14.4mmHg
Abdomen 10%	2 mmHg	3 mmHg	4 mmHg

Garment Wearing Tips

◆ Gradient support stockings are worn during the day, not during sleep. They are designed to move fluids while you are moving.

◆ You should exercise with compression and in moderation. The preferred exercise is walking. Swimming requires no compression, if the affected part is fully submerged. Remember: All other exercises require compression to be worn. After swimming, wash affected area, apply lotions or creams, then apply compression garment.

◆ Skin care – This is very important in order to wear garments longer with greater comfort. Stockings strip the skin of its natural moisture and applying proper lotions and creams replenish moisture. (see *Chapter 5* for more details)

◆ Weight loss – extra body weight puts more pressure on an affected area already compromised. Body fluids do not pass through enlarged fat cells as effectively.

◆ When a bodily injury occurs to an affected area, (especially to the legs, leaving them inflamed, bruised, swollen, or discolored) tests should be done to rule out blood clots.

◆ Diet and fluids – if you are dieting, follow the plan outlined by your dietitian. Gradually increase *water* intake to ½ your weight in ounces of water daily. If traveling by air, add 50% more water. For example, if you weigh 150 lbs., drink 75 ounces of water – add another 37 ½ ounces if you are traveling by air, or 1 1/2 times normal daily intake.

◆ Daily wear – do not sit or stand too long while wearing

gradient support stockings. Move frequently. If sitting, elevate the legs and do leg exercises such as rotating the ankles, flexion/extension of the foot/feet. If standing, bend the knees or stretch out the calf muscle by standing on the toes, walk, etc. *Gradiency* means most compression at the farthest point, wrist or ankle, and gradually decreasing up the limb. Sitting with knees bent at 90 degrees for an extended period of time without exercise will move fluids into the knee. The characteristic of gradient compression is it will always move fluids up the limb, and a bend in the limb inhibits fluids from moving past that bend. The same applies to an affected arm when compression is applied. Exercises for the arm include: flexion/extension, and rotation of the wrist.

♦ Daily care — when a garment is first purchased or worn, apply the date on the garment band with an indelible marking pen. This will denote the age of the garment, alerting you to the time for purchase of a new one. If you have 1 garment, wearing and washing it daily, it will last about 3 months. Ideally, it is best to have a least 2 garments you can rotate. These will last about 6+ months, provided every time they are worn, they are washed. Washing not only removes bodily wastes that have been absorbed into the garment fibers, it also returns the garment to its former elasticity. It has been proven that lack of proper care of garments, deteriorates the elastic fibers causing them to wear out more readily. When garments wear out, the affected area will begin to show signs of increased swelling. Garments must be compatible with the lymphedema condition to maintain reduction.

♦ Classes of Compression (CC) – medical gradient compression garments:

CCI = 20–30 mmHg pressure beginning at ankle or wrist
CCII = 30–40mmHg pressure beginning at ankle or wrist
CCIII = 40–50 mmHg pressure beginning at ankle or wrist
CCIV = above 50 mmHg pressure beginning at the ankle

♦ Air travel or increased altitudes – if a specific compression class is being worn on a daily basis, it will be necessary to either purchase a garment with a higher compression class, or apply short-stretch bandages over the existing garment. Affected areas already requiring compression are further compromised by air travel and increased altitudes. The body swells more in these conditions and will need additional pressure or a higher compression class. For example, if you are wearing a CCI garment daily, a compression class II will be needed for air travel or increased altitudes.

♦ *Anti-Emboli* stockings – usually worn during surgery and a short time post-op. Their purpose is to prevent pooling of blood and move body fluids during rest, thus preventing blood clots. These move fluids when the body is at rest.

♦ For high fashion – try wearing a pair of plain or fashion nylons over a skin-tone gradient compression stocking. The compression stockings become "invisible," and the outer more fashionable stockings look "smashing." Fashion stockings come in a variety of colors and textures and create a wonderful illusion over compression stockings. **The key is to get creative.**

Compression Gloves

When a compression sleeve is fit for the first time, it has been our experience that wearing the sleeve daily for one week will be sufficient to reduce swelling in the hand. However, if it does not and the hand becomes more swollen, purchase an *Isotoner*-type glove. Remove the leather strips, then apply the glove on the hand while wearing the sleeve. In most instances, this will relieve the hand of some swelling. If wearing the sleeve and Isotoner-type glove daily for a week does not significantly reduce the hand, contact your lymphedema specialist for further instructions on compression therapy.

Maintenance Phase

Daily Routine
When Wearing Compression Garments

Morning:

♦ Wash affected area/areas, rinse and dry thoroughly.

♦ Apply *Lymphoderm* Lotion.

♦ Apply A&D Ointment to:

    – toes/feet & back of knee (leg affected)

    – fingers/hand up to elbow crease (arm affected)

♦ Apply *A lps* Lotion to:
    – toes/feet up to knee (leg affected)
    – finger/hand up to elbow crease (arm affected)

♦ Apply garment (stocking or sleeve).

♦ If needed, apply *Skin A dhesive* on skin at level of top band – do not apply to inner leg near groin or on inner arm near armpit.

Evening:

- Remove garment.

- Wash affected area or areas.

- Wash garment in warm mild soapy water, rinse well, towel dry and hang overnight on hanger.

- Apply *Lymphoderm* Lotion to affected area/areas.

- Retire for the night without compression unless otherwise directed.

Note:
Good maintenance in lymphedema care may
never result in total reduction equal to unaffected area.
However. good maintenance may result in having soft
tissue, staying infection-free, and having good, healthy
skin.

Chapter 5

Skin Care

The skin is the largest organ of the body, and it requires as much attention as any other organ. It is 15% of the total body weight. Properties of the skin are: it is the principle seat of the sense of touch; it may be regarded as the covering for protecting the deeper tissues; it plays an important part in the regulation of body temperature; and it is an absorbing and excretory organ. As an excretory organ, the skin has its own natural moisturizers, secreting sweat and sebum, and it has tiny pores through which wastes from underlying tissues can escape. The skin "breathes," that is, it takes in oxygen and discharges carbon dioxide. These pores, or "openings" in the skin, cover the **epidermis**, the top layer of the skin, and are more numerous in some areas of the body than in others. Pores allow absorption of many substances, such as: special drugs, chemicals, creams, lotions or ointments which combat infection, condition the skin, and overcome or prevent dryness.

The **subcutaneous** layer of the skin is the protective layer for the outer skin. It gives contour and smoothness to the body, stores fat for body energy, and contains a network of arteries and lymphatics. It is here in the "ground substance" where the blood and lymph supply nourishment to the tissues, and where the exchange of waste products from the cells takes place.

The pores of the epidermis excrete wastes from the underlying subcutaneous layer. Gradient compression garments, which are worn on an affected lymphedema limb already filled with lymph and waste products, can absorb this residue. In addition, these garments also "hug" the affected part and absorb the skin's natural moisture, sweat, and sebum. And, when this "protective mantle" of the skin is lost, the skin becomes dry and loses its natural ability to self protect, leaving it exposed to negative environmental conditions. In addition, the already-compromised lymphedema situation with extra wastes and lymph in the subcutaneous layer causes further changes in the skin. Over a period of time, if the skin is not given proper treatment, infections such as *cellulitis* may be a real problem.

Proper protective skin care for an affected body part:

♦ Wash the affected area with a mild antibacterial soap. To remove any dryness of the skin, use a soft nylon "puff ball," and go over the area lightly to *exfoliate*. This procedure smoothes and softens the skin preparing it to better receive water-base creams or lotions.

♦ Rinse the skin very well and dry thoroughly. Apply a water-base cream or lotion, e.g., *Lymphoderm* lotion. *Be sure to always do a skin test of any new product before fully applying it. This will help you identify if you have an allergic reaction to the product.*

♦ Always apply the lotions or creams in the direction into which fluids are being moved during self-MLD. Your lymphedema specialist will set up protocol for self-MLD according to your specific needs.

♦ A small amount of A&D ointment in the creases and folds will decrease the "rubber band" effect at the elbow, wrist, ankle, or back of knee. Be careful not to use too much ointment, as ointments will not only cause a "dragging" effect upon pulling up the garment, but also petroleum products tend to break down elastic fibers in a gradient compression garment.

90

- Use donning aids such as: *Alps* silicon lotion, slippeze, *Elfie*, and other donning accessories. *Alps* lotion is a water-base silicon lotion, is hypoallergenic, serves as a barrier between the skin and the garment, and can be applied over existing moisturizers, trapping them next to the skin. This allows you to wear gradient compression garments for longer periods of time more comfortably.

The skin will reflect the quality of health of the underlying tissues. If the tissues are full of waste products and residual fluids, the skin will not be nourished and will show dramatic signs of change. It is also very important to incorporate the basics of good diet, positive attitude, and exercise in your daily skin regimen. Positive results will follow (wellness in mind, body, and spirit) and the skin will show it. The more frequently skin care is done, the skin will become softer and more pliable. The result is that the skin will require less cream or lotion. **Remember: Always wash the skin and apply lotions or creams before applying any garment, and again after removing the garment at the end of each day.**

Shaving – An electric razor is recommended. If a depilatory is to be used (e.g., *Neat*), always test the product on the skin before using the product. Razor blades are not recommended, as they may nick the skin bringing about an increased chance for infection. Consult your lymphedema specialist if you have questions about shaving or any negative effects after shaving.

Massage – Massage is good, but should be performed only by a certified massage therapist who is highly qualified to do body massage. *Massaging the affected quadrant is not advised,* as it may complicate the lymphedema condition cause more swelling. Your massage therapist can, however, massage other areas of the body.

Nail Care – Retain the services of a highly qualified manicurist for nail care. Sanitized supplies should be used. It is best to purchase your own polishes and equipment and have your manicurist apply them during nail care services. This avoids any cross-contamination. If you notice a hangnail or other imperfection on the nails, consult your lymphedema therapist for advice. Trauma to nails has been a source of infection for a lymphedema limb.

Daily Routine When Wearing Compression Garments

Morning:

♦ Wash affected area/areas, rinse, pat excess water leaving skin slightly moist.

♦ Apply lotion to affected area/areas.

♦ Apply A&D Ointment to:
  — back of knee (leg affected)
  — elbow crease (arm affected)

♦ Apply *A lps* Lotion to:
  — toes/feet up to knee (leg affected)
  — fingers/hand up to elbow crease (arm affected)

♦ Apply garment (stocking or sleeve) with rubber gloves on hands, using pads of fingers so as not to snag or pull holes in garment.

♦ Apply Skin Adhesive on skin at level of top band. Do not apply to inner leg near groin or in armpit. (Skin adhesive is not used if garment has silicone band at top.)

Evening:

- Remove garment.
- Wash affected area/areas, rinse, pat excess water, leaving skin slightly moist.
- Apply lotion to affected area/areas. Apply A&D Ointment to feet/hand.
- Wash garment in warm mild soap (*Dreft* or *Ivory*), rinse well. Roll garment in thick fluffy towel to remove excess moisture and hang to dry overnight.
- Go to sleep without compression, unless otherwise directed.

Note*:* One stocking worn daily will last 3-4 months. Replace them every 3-4 months to control swelling.

- **Always exercise with compression unless water exercises are performed.**
- **Increase compression if you vacation or air travel at over 4,000 ft. elevation or higher.**
- **Always exercise with compression unless water exercises are performed.**
- **1st day garment is worn, mark the date on inside of band with a permanent marker.**

Treat Lymphedema Skin As a Wound

Since waste fluids exist just under the surface of the skin, the skin is not healthy. We already know that "old skin" is sloughed every 28-30 days and "new skin" comes from healthy tissues of the subcutaneous layer, just under the surface of the skin. So, we can conclude that the skin cannot be healthy if the underlying tissues are not healthy.

Steps in Caring for Lymphedema Skin

1. **Cleanse** - wash with mild soap, rinse, remove excess water.

2. **Treat** - while skin is still moist, apply a water-base cream.

3. **Protect** - apply special creams & pads to open or traumatized areas before donning gradient compression garments.

This should be done in the AM before donning garments and in the PM after removing garments.

Daily Skin Care For Very Dry Skin

Morning:
♦ Soak area in *warm* lightly soapy water (table salt may be substituted) — 20 minutes.

♦ While soaking feet and/or hands, wiggle appendages in water while *lightly* running soft wash cloth over the area to remove dead skin (*exfoliate*).

♦ Rinse well and pat excess water with soft towel

♦ While skin is still moist, apply EUCERIN or a light water base lotion to areas especially between toes and fingers making sure all lotion is absorbed

♦ Apply A/D Ointment all over toes & feet – cover with plastic bag or seran wrap – hold in place with cotton socks – leave on until next soaking.

Noon: Repeat Morning Directions

Evening:
♦ Repeat AM directions

♦ To affected area, apply emollient A/D ointment thoroughly, wrap feet/ hands in saran wrap, and cover with soft cotton socks. **Sleep in this over night.**

You will see much healthier skin after applying this intensive skin care regimen for one week.

Chapter 6

Exercise

During Intensive Combined Decongestive Therapy (CDT), when there is gradient bandaging 23/7, each patient, while bandaged, is instructed in lymphedema-specific exercises. Following CDT, a lymphedema specialist should be consulted before commencing any weight lifting program. Most generally, lifting anything over 10 lbs. may cause negative effects on an affected area. Here is a good guideline to follow when monitoring lymphedema: When performing any task or exercise, use the **"cause and effect" rule** — whatever you do, check the effects on the affected area. Each lymphedema case is different and each person affected will react differently. If the lymphedema condition worsens after performing a task or a specific exercise, reassess what you are doing and how it is being done. **Remember: Moderation is the Key.**

The weight you are carrying may be too heavy, or the task may be too strenuous. Consult with a lymphedema specialist for guidance and direction concerning your individual exercise routine.

Swimming is one of the best all-around exercises. The water automatically gives gradient pressure, as long as the affected limb is totally submerged while swimming. If you were to stand in water to just above your waist, you would receive approximately 35-mmHg pressure at your knees. This is class 2 compression (30-40mmHg pressure). Therefore, swimming does not require compression. However, following swimming, it is important to wash the affected area, apply lotions, and then apply a clean gradient compression garment to the affected area.

Walking is the "ultimate-weapon" exercise, since it uses almost all of the body's 650 muscles and 206 bones without stressing the body. Also, those bones and muscles are used in a more balanced way than in any other exercise. It is the most effective exercise for weight control because it can be performed every day, by every "body," for long periods of time throughout one's life. Walking, as well as any other exercise, requires proper shoes and equipment before commencing.

Yoga is also very good. It strengthens muscles and joints, reduces tension, and relaxes the whole body. It is best to begin slowly and build your regimen as the body can tolerate. Always remember the **"cause and effect"** rule.

Abdominal/diaphragm breathing *(Deep breathing)* – Practice pushing air into your "belly" or abdomen when you breathe in, count to 7 while inhaling, hold your breath to the count of 7, then to the count of 7 slowly release your breath while the abdomen flattens. Repeat this 10 times until you can build to 25 or more times/day. This is very relaxing before bedtime and usually sleep comes before completing the exercise. Deep breathing also clears the lungs and brings oxygen to all the tissues.

Exercise is the "indispensable ingredient" for a positive correlation between doing better and feeling better. Through the ages, human beings have recognized that physical condition and emotional well-being are linked. It takes about one hour/day for a good exercise program and the only way to work exercise into your life is to remove some "dead weight" from your schedule. **Make a commitment to exercise.**

Try a "FIT" program:
Frequency (how often)
Intensity (how hard)
Time (how long)

The only way to fail is not to participate. For lymphedema, any exercise, with the exception of swimming, requires compression . Muscular action with compression moves fluids more efficiently. Without compression the affected part will become more swollen.

Exercises for Patients with Arm Lymphedema
(Apply gradient compression garment):

Each exercise should be repeated 10x with appropriate pauses while bandaged or wearing gradient compression garment. Repeat exercises 2-3x per day and never over exert. Exhale while contracting, inhale while relaxing. Breathing exercises can be interspersed in the breaks.

1. Position: Sitting
   Procedure: Place the hands flat on the table. Raise the hand against an imagined resistance and lower it again. Press the hand into the table. Be careful not to raise the wrist fully in extension.

2. Position: Sitting
   Procedure: Lay the forearms on the table and circle the hands against an imagined resistance.

3. Position: Sitting
   Procedure: With the forearms on the table and the fingers outstretched and extended, slowly close the hands to a fist then open again,

stretching and extending the fingers.

4. Position: Sitting
   Procedure: With the arms hanging at the sides, raise them to 90-degree with the fingers outstretched and extended. Close the hand to a fist against an imagined resistance. Supinate (palms up) the arms and bend at the elbow (no more than 80-degrees) against an imagined resistance then straighten them while stretching and extending the fingers.

5. Position: Sitting
   Procedure: Raise the arms from the sides with the elbows slightly flexed. Press the hands together in front of the body (hold for 7 seconds). With the fingers interlocked, try to pull the hands apart (hold for 7 seconds).

6. Position: Sitting
   Procedure: Raise the arms in pronation (palms down) to 90-degrees with the fingers outstretched and extended. Supinate the hands against an imagined resistance.

7. Position: Sitting
   Procedure: Raise and lower the shoulders, then make circles forwards and backwards.

Remember: Always exercise with compression unless you are doing water exercises.

Exercises for Patients with Leg Lymphedema
(*Apply compression garment*):

Each exercise should be repeated 10x with appropriate pauses while bandaged or wearing gradient compression garment. Repeat exercises 2-3x per day and never overexert. **Exhale while contracting, inhale while relaxing.** Breathing exercises can be interspersed during breaks.

1. Position: Standing
   Procedure: "Roll on the soles" — change position from heel to toes.

2. Position: Standing
   Procedure: With feet angled out (legs externally rotated), lift one knee until the hip is in 90-degree flexion while pointing the toes down to the floor.

3. Position: Sitting with legs outstretched
   Procedure: Bend the knees then "roll the soles" from heel to toes.

4. Position: Supine (lying on the back)
   Procedure: "Bicycle" with the legs in the air while flexing and extending the ankle. Extend against an imagined resistance.

5. Position: Supine with knees bent
   Procedure: One after the other, extend and hold the right and left legs in the air (please modify if this is difficult). Against an imagined resistance, make circles to the right and to the left with the feet then circle inward, then outwards.

6. Position: *Supine* with knees bent
  Procedure: Raise the head, right shoulder and arm and try to stretch past the left knee. Repeat on the opposite side with the left shoulder and arm.
  Variation: Raiser the upper body and press both knees together (hold for 7 seconds). Repeat while pushing the legs apart.

Note these differences:

ACE bandages or "long stretch bandages" move fluids while you are resting and can be applied directly over the skin.

"Short stretch bandages" move fluids while you are moving or exercising. They are applied gradiently over padding to move fluids from the farthest point of the limb to the nearest.

Chapter 7

Directional Flow Garments (DFG)

Directional flow garments (DFG) are designed to produce
gradient pressure from many angles. Each unit is also
constructed with passive compression to allow movement
of lymph fluid along normal lymph pathways. These three
ingredients — **gradient pressure, directional flow, and
passive compression** — must work together to be
effective. Each garment is fabricated according to patient
specific protocol for therapy. That is, directional flow
channels follow manual lymph drainage treatment protocol
for each individual, moving fluids directionally bypassing
congested areas.

Sewn into channels of these directional flow products are
hundreds of high resistant foam chips of various densities
and sizes. The exterior is 94% polyester and 6% *Lycra*.
Before using the product, it is necessary to become familiar
with your treatment provider's recommended care and
usage suggestions. This will enhance the unit's effective-
ness and longevity.

Directional flow products are not intended to function on a
stand-alone basis. For best results, a DFG should be applied
in one of the following ways and *always* with a
lymphedema specialist's direct supervision or counsel:

- under low-stretch bandaging
- under a gradient sequential pneumatic pump appliance
- under an outer binder or similar product

The following pages explain these different uses in greater
detail.

DFG is used instead of padding under short or low-stretch bandaging.

Because these garments have gradient pressure, directional flow, and padded passive compression, they have been used during the intensive and transitional phases of Combined Decongestive Therapy (CDT). These garments are designed patient-specific, are one-piece in most instances, and afford much easier home self-care during all phases of the care for lymphedema. During the intensive phase of CDT, short-stretch bandages can be applied over the directional flow garment for 23 hrs/day, with one hour off to include other forms of self-care. This treatment plan not only breaks up fibrotic areas more efficiently, but also fluids move more quickly into collateral pathways.

After the intensive phase of CDT is complete, patients progress to a gradient compression garment for daytime use (*daytime garment*) and continue to bandage over their directional flow garment for nighttime or sleeping hours (*nighttime garment*). This seems to be a very good "interim" treatment plan during the transitional phase, because the nighttime garment helps the body to continue to move fluids into collateral pathways while the patient is sleeping or resting for an extended amount of time.

Most often during the maintenance phase of lymphedema care, patients continue to follow this plan for several months. By this time patients have become so familiar with their lymphedema condition and their individual self-care that they are able to use their own judgment about when it becomes necessary to apply the nighttime DFG. The directional flow garment will continue to move fluids during the hours of sleep after the daytime compression garment has been removed.

DFG is used with Gradient Sequential Pump under a pneumatic appliance

A directional flow garment applied under the pneumatic appliance, which is connected to a sequential pump, is designed to move fluids out of an affected limb away from the congested body area. Pumping commences while Manual Lymph Drainage (MLD) is being performed. It works in much the same manner as bandaging except that fluids move much more quickly. Time for treatment is set 30-45 minutes at 40mmHg distal (farthest) chamber, patient specific to tolerance and lymphedema condition. Calibrations are set at: 40mmHg pressure distally, decreasing to 30mmHg proximal pressure, depending upon each individual lymphedema condition. Fluids move very quickly under these conditions. Pump use during home care and treatment should be set and monitored by a lymphedema specialist. If there is a spotty redness lasting more than 10-20 minutes post-treatment, external pressure and/or usage time should be re-evaluated. Discontinue treatment and seek counsel from a lymphedema specialist before commencing therapy.

DFG is used instead of bandaging under a Binder or Outer Jacket

When bandaging becomes a challenge, especially in cases where affected areas are over-sized or areas are misshapen, e.g., chest, abdomen, an elasticized outer jacket or *Velcro* closure binder will be used over the directional flow garment. The patient is able to apply this outer jacket much more easily during home self care. Most binders and outer jackets are custom made to fit each patient's specific needs.

Care — Use a mild detergent that will not damage foam

(read the label). Wash in machine on slow cycle and double rinse to remove any residual soap. Use fast spin cycle to remove excess water. You may dry on air or low heat of your dryer cycle. However, for longer garment life, line drying is best. Use of a fan or blow dryer will reduce drying time. Do not dry with high heat. The DFG should be thoroughly dry during an 8-hour period in order to avoid developing mold spores. If the unit does not feel completely dry after 8 hours, turn the garment inside out, place it in a lingerie bag or pillowcase, and put in automatic dryer's air-dry cycle until completely dry. To reduce the number of washings and extend unit longevity, it is recommended that a clean cotton stockinette be applied to the limb before applying the DFG. If worn daily, the DFG should be laundered once a week.

Application — Before wearing the unit, ensure that the seams are on the outside so as not to compromise/irritate the skin's integrity. The "outside" of the unit also has a manufacturer's tag attached along the inside seam. For arms and legs, gently roll back the top of the unit, inside out and half the length of the unit. Apply to limb by pulling back the top (inside out) portion. Take the unit off by again gently rolling the top of the unit down half-way and pull arm/leg out. Use rubber gloves when applying the DFG to avoid having fingernails tear the material. Pulling too hard, fast, and aggressively while applying the unit or removing it could damage the unit and/or decrease its longevity. Improper use and care will void the warranty. Each unit is meant to last several months or longer, relative to usage and care. Materials and workmanship are warranted if shown to be defective when received, or if there is an error in meeting the specified measurements as provided by the therapist or authorized reseller.

Nine Steps For Applying Directional Flow Garments (DFG)

1

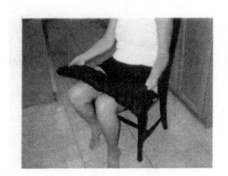

2

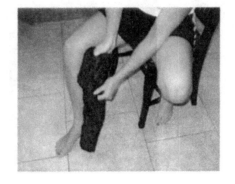

3

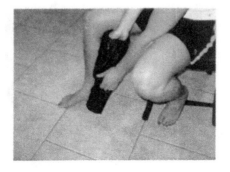

4

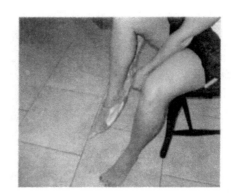

5

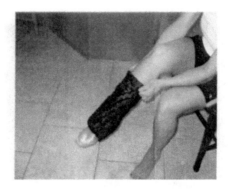

6

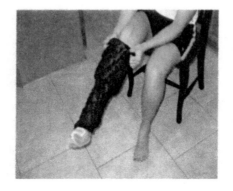

7

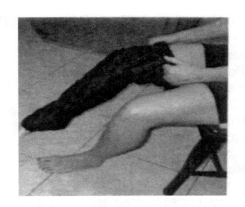

8

9

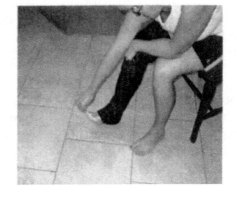

110

Use of Directional Flow Garment (DFG)

Indications:
- Primary or secondary lymphedema
- Radiation fibrosis

Contraindications:
- Active infection
- Fever
- Renal Disease or Impairment
- Congestive heart failure
- Known or suspected deep vein thrombosis or thrombophlebitis

Suggested Use With Gradient Sequential Pump — The DFG is applied under a pump sleeve and pumping commences while MLD is being performed. Time of use under the pump is 1-hour maximum, not to exceed 40mmHg pressure, distally (most pressure beginning on foot or hand).

Calibrations should be set at: 40mmHg pressure distally, decreasing to 30mmHg proximal pressure. Fluids move very quickly under these conditions. Pump use during home care and treatment should be set and monitored by a lymphedema specialist. If there is spotty redness lasting more than 10 – 20 minutes post-treatment, external pressure and/or usage time should be re-evaluated. Discontinue treatment and seek counsel from a lymphedema specialist before commencing therapy.

Types and Styles — DFG are designed for any body part and the specific needs of each patient. The lymphedema specialist sets protocol for therapy and DFG garments are designed accordingly.

Custom DFG for Every Body Part

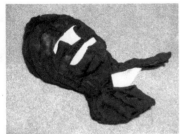

Full Head, Neck and Face
Compression

Chest/Torso Vest
with arm attached

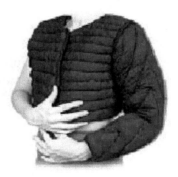

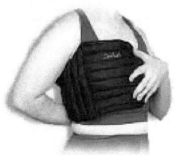

Unilateral Breast/Torso
Compression Wrap

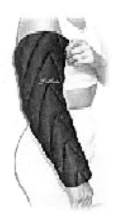

Arm Unit—
Wrist to axilla

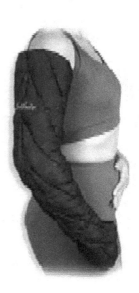

Full Arm Unit—
Finger tips to axilla

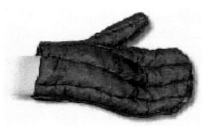

Hand Mitt

Abdominal/Shorts Unit

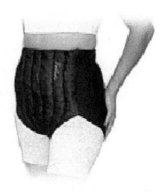

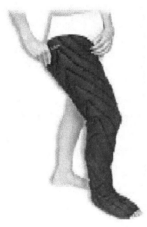

Full Leg Unit —
Toes to groin with hip riser

"Chaps-style"—
Full Leg with waist and hip attachment

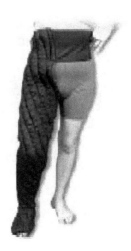

Chapter 8

Pumps

Gradient & Sequential Pressure

Sequential pumps with calibrated gradient pressure can be very effective in home care maintenance of lymphedema, provided they are used under strict supervision and guidance by a lymphedema specialist. When pumps are used for home maintenance of lymphedema, the lymphedema specialist: sets the correct calibrations on the pump specific to each lymphedema case; teaches the patient about the pump and how to use it; measures and fits the directional flow garment that must be worn under the pump sleeve; instructs the patient in the care of the skin during and after pumping; teaches when and how to apply both daytime and nighttime garments (DFG); and gives specific details concerning protocol for pump therapy and Manual Lymph Drainage (MLD). **Note: Never use a pump without proper instructions from a lymphedema specialist.**

Gradient pressure – Pump is set manually so that most pressure is at the farthest point on the limb, gradually decreasing up the limb. For example, the first chamber may be set at 40mmHg pressure at the wrist or ankle, gradually decreasing to 30mmHg pressure at the armpit (axilla) or groin, depending upon the number of chambers each pump has. Gradiency is set specific to each lymphedema case. Some pumps automatically calibrate gradiently once the first chamber is set by the lymphedema specialist. If this is not a pump feature, the lymphedema specialist must set each chamber specific to each patient's needs.

Sequential pressure – Once the pressure is set gradiently, each chamber inflates to capacity beginning with the first chamber at the farthest point on the limb until all chambers in sequence up the limb are fully inflated. This is known as the *inflation cycle*. The *deflation cycle* begins when each chamber, beginning with the firstchamber at the farthest point, deflates in sequence up the limb until all chambers are fully deflated. Cycle times and number of chambers differ with each pump.

When ordering a pump for home use, order a segmental home model with calibrated pressure. A segmental gradient pressure pneumatic appliance must also be ordered with the pump. This is the pump sleeve that is applied on the affected limb and has tubing, which is connected to the pump for airflow. In addition, it is advised that a directional flow garment be applied on the affected limb prior to the pump sleeve or pneumatic appliance. We have found that this is the safest way to use the pump. Use of a gradient sequential pump with a directional flow garment produces gradient and sequential pumping, while the directional flow garment moves lymph into collateral pathways, by-passing congested areas. Pumping in this manner moves fluids very rapidly and is usually applied for 60 minutes each session, while Manual Lymph Drainage is opening collateral pathways. Patients using pumps for home care usually set aside time of treatment in the evening before going to bed because of the treatment's relaxing effects. This also enhances removal of any excess fluids remaining in body tissues at the end of the day.

Recommended Use of Pumps:
- Primary and secondary lymphedema
- Venous and lymphatic insufficiency
- Post traumatic, Post paralytic and other edemas
- Wound Healing

116

Contraindications for Pump Use:
- Presence of pain or numbness in the extremity
- Severe arteriosclerosis or other ischemic vascular diseases
- Massive edema of the legs or arms due to congestive heart failure or pulmonary edema
- Extreme deformity of the limbs
- Known or suspected deep vein thrombosis or thrombophlebitis
- Pulmonary embolism
- Presence of gangrene
- Dermatitis
- Untreated or infected wounds
- Recent skin grafts
- Acute infection not yet treated with antibiotic therapy

Stanford University Study

In 2002, Stanley Rockson, MD and his Stanford University colleagues, Andrzej Szuba, MD, PhD, and Radha Achalu, MD, completed a clinical study proving the safety and efficacy of gradient, sequential, *Intermittent Pneumatic Compression* (IPC) for the treatment of lymphedema associated with breast cancer.

Report of Stanford findings:

1. Intermittent Pneumatic Compression (IPC), added to other elements of decongestive lymphatic therapy, enhances the treatment of lymphedema associated with axillary lymph node dissection in breast cancer patients.
2. Lymphedema of the arm is a common aftermath of breast cancer treatment with surgery and radiation. The condition is debilitating, physically and psychologically, and treatment options are quite limited.

3. The use of pneumatic compression pumps as a potential treatment has fallen into disfavor because of old, poorly substantiated claims that the use of pumps can actually create more problems than they solve.

4. This study is the first prospective evaluation of the use of these pumps as adjunctive therapy to the existing physiotherapies for breast cancer lymphedema, both in acute and maintenance management. Both were evaluated for efficacy and the potential for creating side effects.

5. Overall, combined decongestive therapy (CDT) resulted in a mean volume reduction of 45.3% compared with 26% for decongestive lymphatic therapy. IPC resulted in a reduction of mean volume of 89.5ml compared with an increase of 32.7ml with decongestive lymphatic therapy alone.

6. The study documented efficacy in both acute and chro ic maintenance, when added to conventional measures. There was no evidence that the therapy created complications in the skin or the joints as previously alleged.

Conclusion: Intermittant Pneumatic Compression (IPC) was found to be a very safe and cost-efficient method of treatment that has been inappropriately neglected and may actually be a very effective way to improve the well-being of a large number of patients with this common disease.

Chapter 9

Positive Steps to Wellness

On his birthday, a well-known celebrity asked his father what was the secret to a long, happy, and healthy life. His father replied that he always tried to have three positive things going on in his life. They were: *someone to love, something to do, and something to look forward to.*

We have long heard about the "mind-body connection" – what we think, usually happens. Positive thinking brings about positive effects and, conversely, negative thinking, negative effects. The way we think can result in our lives being a "living heaven" or a suffering hell." We can choose which way we want our lives to go. Life is not — and was never said to be — a "bed of roses," but cultivating a positive thought pattern daily can turn our "lemons into lemonade" and make a smiling countenance.

Wellness is being totally whole. A whole person is made up of many parts: spiritual, physical, emotional, mental, social, and intellectual. To achieve wellness we must seek to become a whole being by developing all the parts. The whole is only as good as its parts, and the parts only as good as the whole. When something occurs affecting the body or any part of the body, it is most often the result of a negative happening. If we were to reflect on our lives, a severe illness usually followed a very critical time in our life.

It takes a lot of effort to be positive, especially when life does not always "deal out a good hand." If we take the "one -day-at-a-time" philosophy while working at it, eventually great changes will unfold in our lives. Here are some *positive* tips:

Methods of Relaxation:

Physical:

Start a daily exercise routine with low impact — walking, cycling, swimming, Yoga, planned exercise for lymphedema with compression. Except for swimming, always do these in moderation with compression.

♦ **Deep Breathing** – Diaphragmatic breathing several times/day and also while exercising.

♦ **Good Posture** – The added weight of a heavy limb/ limbs can throw the body off balance. Look at body basics: good shoes and support such as orthotics, support socks and hosiery, foot care.

♦ **Skin Care** – The use of essential oils blended with certain creams and oils mixed in appropriate amounts can soothe dry, cracked hands and feet. Essential oils such as lavender, chamomile, clary sage, peppermint, tea tree, and lemongrass blended with an appropriate cream will not only heal and fight infection, but also serve as a pleasant, therapeutic inhalant. For a soothing hand or foot care recipe: add 3-5 drops of an essential oil per tablespoon of cream or oil. Apply on affected part, working in well, then apply a soft cotton glove or sock – leave on all night.

♦ **Facials** – Applications specific for each skin type not only can be beneficial for the face but also entirely relaxing for the body. Looking Good Makes You Feel Good!

♦ **Manicures and Foot Care** – Secure the services of a professional who uses very clean techniques and instruments. Infections can begin in unsanitary conditions. More severe chronic conditions such as diabetes, venous insufficiency, venous ulcers, or arterial problems: consult a physician or podiatrist.

♦ **Body Massage** – Caution should be used not to massage the affected part.

♦ **Whirlpool Baths** – Very good if the water temperature is not too hot.

♦ **Dietary Needs** – Our soil no longer provides us with food to supply optimum nutrition for body cell replacement. Though it is very important to have a well-rounded daily diet, nutritional supplements have become a necessary part of our diet in order to supply our bodies with micronutrients we can no longer receive from the food we eat. In addition, our generation is exposed to more emotional stress, pollutants, toxins, radiation, and drugs than any other generation. This is the main reason we are seeing more chronic degenerative diseases affecting persons at a much younger age. We must build up our antioxidant defense systems to optimum levels. The tables on the following two pages detail a daily food plan and a complete list of antioxidants:

Dietary Guidelines

Based on the new guidelines, here is what the average American is supposed to eat on a given day:

6-11 Servings of **Bread, Cereal, Rice and Pasta**
    1 serving = 1 slice bread or 1/2 cup cooked rice

2-4 Servings of **Fruit**
    1 serving = 1 medium fruit or 4oz. fresh fruit juice

3-5 Servings of **Vegetables**
    1 serving = 1 cup raw, leafy vegetables or 6oz. vegetable juice

2-3 Servings of **Dairy Foods**
    1 serving = 1 cup yogurt or 1 cup milk or 1oz. cheese

2-3 Servings of **Meat, Fish, Poultry, Dry Beans, Eggs and Nuts**
    1 serving = 3 to 4oz **animal protein**, roughly the size of a deck of cards, or 1/4 cup nuts

Fats (at the very top of the Food Guide Pyramid,) are to be used sparingly.

Experts agree that roughly 55-60% of food should be in the form of carbohydrates (grains, starches, fruit, and vegetables). Fats should constitute no more than 30% of daily calories (the average intake in the United States is around 37%). Protein consumption should be limited, which will happen naturally if you watch your portion size of protein-rich foods, such as meat. Most Americans eat more than 100 grams of protein daily — twice as much as they actually need.

Salt intake should be limited to 2400mg daily. This can be achieved by avoiding highly salted food and not adding additional salt to food.

Antioxidants

Vitamin A	It is recommended that patients avoid taking straight vitamin A. Supplementation of beta-carotene can be used instead of vitamin A.
Beta-carotene	15,000 to 25,000 IU daily
Vitamin C	1 to 2 grams daily
Vitamin E	400 to 600 IU daily a d-alpha-tocopherol
Glutathione	10 to 20 mg daily
N-acetyl-L-cysteine	60 to 75 mg daily
Alpha lipoic acid	15 to 20 mg daily
Coenzyme Q10	15 to 30 mg daily
Bioflavonoid	It is recommended to take a combination of several complex bioflavonoids, which should include rutin, cruciferous, bilberry extract, green tea extract, broccoli concentrate and quercetin; other combinations may also be effective.

Vitamin B Complex:

Vitamin B1 (Thiamin)	20 to 30 mg daily
Vitamin B2 (Riboflavin)	25 to 35 mg daily
Vitamin B3 (Niacin)	40 to 50 mg daily
Vitamin B5 (Pantothenic acid)	90 to 120 mg daily
Vitamin B6 (Pyridoxine)	20 to 30 mg daily
Vitamin B12 (Cobalamin)	50 to 100 mg daily
Folic Acid	1000 mcg daily
Choline	100 to 125 mg daily
Inositol	100 to 200 mg daily

Other Vitamins:

Vitamin D	500 to 800 IU daily as vitamin D3 (cholecalciferol)
Vitamin K	50 to 100 mcg daily

Minerals:

Calcium	800 to 1500 mg daily as calcium citrate
Magnesium	500 to 800 mg daily
Zinc	20 to 30 mg daily as zinc picolinate or chelated zinc

This level of supplementation has been shown in medical literature to be effective and safe in properly nourishing body cells at an optimum level. The health benefits that are received using this supplemental program are:

- A decrease in risk of cardiovascular disease (stroke, heart attack, and hardening of the arteries in general), LDL is reduced
- A decrease in the risk of developing cancer
- Improvement in the immune system
- A decrease in the risk of age-related cataract formation and the development of age-related macular degeneration
- Hopefully, a decrease in the risk of Alzheimer's dementia, Parkinson's disease, rheumatoid arthritis, osteoarthritis, Crohn's disease, and all the other degenerative diseases that are now found to be the cause of oxidative stress
- Hopefully, an improvement in asthma and the progression of emphysema
- Hopefully, a decrease in the development of diabetes
- Hopefully, the progression of osteoporosis slows and is prevented

This program is not a treatment for disease. Rather, it is a way to build our own antioxidant defense system and our own immune system. A healthy body is our best defense against developing a chronic degenerative disease and cancer. *Give the body what it needs and it will have the capability to heal itself.*

Emotional:

Stress Hurts! — Whenever hopelessness, helplessness, and defeat exist, stress happens. Some people use eating as a way of coping with stress. As the level of stress increases, so does their amount and frequency of food intake increase. It is important to recognize "why you are eating" and then **Get Moving.** Exercise reduces cholesterol and increases muscle capacity. When exercise is lacking, the muscle loses its capability to burn fat. The stress/fat cycle is dependent upon the mind, mouth, and muscle:

+ **Mind:** Identify your stress triggers and define what you do as a result – know what you are feeling.
+ **Mouth:** Monitor what you put into your mouth.
+ **Muscle: Get Moving.** Exercise to burn fat and increase muscle capacity.

Continued stress can result in increased anger. Extreme, unusual, or long lasting stress increases blood cholesterol levels, and can increase anger, blood pressure, and heart rate. Over a long period of stress, the arteries become affected, resulting in immune system deficiencies, increased risk of heart attacks and strokes, exhaustion, and a high risk of developing debilitating disease.

We have already talked about the importance of exercise in not only relieving physical problems, but also reducing the effects of stress during an emotional crisis. Movement therapy and exercises are part of combined decongestive therapy and are necessary to maintain successful results in the treatment of lymphedema. Muscle activity as well as joint movement exerts a profound influence on the lymphatic system. Guidelines for movement therapy are:

+ Individual exercises should not induce pain or

discomfort.
- Jerking, lurching, or straining is not allowed.
- Exercises should not be too stressful nor should they lead to any muscle stiffness.
- Every active phase (maximum 5 seconds) should be followed by a break of equal duration (5 seconds).
- During arm or leg movements, the arm or leg respectively should be kept elevated.

A Few Tips:
- Do your exercises on the floor if at all possible – the bed is too soft.
- Begin with a few exercises only, and then gradually increase the range.
- Do your exercises daily, even twice daily if possible.
- Total time for exercising should not exceed 20 minutes.
- Exercise with compression to intensify lymphatic activity.
- Begin every exercise session with exercises for relaxation and loosening-up.

One of the most powerful ways to decrease stress and increase energy in the body is by breathing with the diaphragm. Learning to calm the mind as well as the body is extremely important in relieving stress. In addition to addressing negative coping patterns, here are some key dietary recommendations:
- Eliminate or restrict the intake of caffeine.
- Eliminate or restrict the intake of alcohol.
- Eliminate refined carbohydrates from the diet.
- Increase the potassium-to-sodium ratio in the diet.
- Eat regular planned meals in a relaxed environment.
- Control food allergies.
- Water (minimum daily intake) divide body weight by 2 = ounces of water/day. For example, if your weight is 150 lbs, you should be drinking a minimum of 75

ounces of water/day. Any fluids in addition to this amount of water is a bonus.

Many people are not aware of what is causing them stress, but they do notice the physical signs of stress: insomnia, depression, fatigue, headache, upset stomach, digestive disturbances, and irritability. The initial body response to stress is "fight-or-flight," designed to counteract danger by mobilizing the body's resources for immediate physical activity. Blood is shunted away from the skin and internal organs, except the heart and lungs, while the amount of blood supplying needed oxygen and glucose to the muscles and brain is increased. Production of digestive secretions is severely reduced since digestive activity is not critical for counteracting stress. It is not the stressor that determines the response; instead it is the individual's internal reaction that triggers the response. The same stress that makes one person sick can be an invigorating experience for another.

Comprehensive stress management involves:
♦ Identify stressors.
♦ Eliminate or reduce sources of stress.
♦ Identify negative coping patterns and replace them with positive ones.
♦ Perform a relaxation/breathing exercise for a minimum of five (5) minutes twice daily.
♦ Manage time effectively.
♦ Enhance relationships through better communication.
♦ Get regular exercise.
♦ Integrate techniques to calm the mind and promote a positive mental attitude.
♦ Follow a healthy diet designed to nourish the body and support physiological processes.

Conditions Linked to Stress	Negative Coping Patterns
Angina	Alcohol
Asthma	Chemical dependence
Autoimmune disease	Drugs - legal and illicit
Cancer	Emotional outbursts
Cardiovascular disease	Excessive behavior
Common cold	Feelings of helplessness
Depression	Irritable bowel
Diabetes (adult onset, Type II)	syndrome
Headaches	Overeating
Hypertension	Overspending
Immune suppression	Premenstrual tension
Rheumatoid arthritis	syndrome
Ulcerative colitis	Smoking
Ulcers	Watching too much TV

Table 1 — Stress Response vs. the Relaxation Response

Stress	Relaxation
The heart rate & force of contraction of heart increases to provide blood to areas necessary for response to the stressful situation.	The heart rate is reduced & the heart beats more effectively. Blood pressure is reduced.
Blood is shunted away from the skin & internal organs, except the heart & lungs, while at the same time the amount of blood supplying needed oxygen & glucose to the muscles & brain is increased.	Blood is shunted towards internal organs, especially those organs involved in digestion.
The rate of breathing increases to supply necessary oxygen to the heart, brain and exercising muscle.	The rate of breathing decreases as oxygen demand is reduced during periods of rest.
Sweat production increases to eliminate toxic compounds produced by the body and to lower body temperature.	Sweat production decreases, as a person who is calm and relaxed does not experience nervous perspiration.
Production of digestive secretions is severely reduced, since digestive activity is not critical for counteracting stress.	Production of digestive secretions is increased, greatly improving digestion.
Blood sugar levels are increased dramatically as the liver dumps stored glucose into the bloodstream.	Blood sugar levels are maintained in the normal physiological range.

Table 2 — Social Readjustment Rating Scale

Rank	Life Event	Mean Value
1	Death of spouse	100
2	Divorce	73
3	Marital separation	65
4	Jail term	63
5	Death of a close family member	63
6	Personal injury or illness	53
7	Marriage	50
8	Fired at work	47
9	Marital reconciliation	45
10	Retirement	45
11	Change in health of family member	44
12	Pregnancy	40
13	Sex difficulties	39
14	Gain of a new family member	39
15	Business adjustment	39
16	Change in financial state	38
17	Death of a close friend	37
18	Change to a different line of work	36
19	Change in number of arguments with spouse	35
20	Large mortgage	31
21	Foreclosure of mortgage or loan	30
22	Change in responsibilities at work	29
23	Son or daughter leaving home	29
24	Trouble with in-laws	29
25	Outstanding personal achievement	28
26	Wife begins or stops work	26
27	Begin or end school	26
28	Change in living conditions	25
29	Revision of personal habits	24
30	Trouble with boss	23
31	Change in work hours or conditions	20
32	Change in residence	20
33	Change in schools	20
34	Change in recreation	19
35	Change in church activities	19
36	Change in social activities	18

Table 2 *continued.*

Rank	Life Event	Mean Value
37	Small mortgage	17
38	Change in sleeping habits	16
39	Change in number of family get-togethers	15
40	Change in eating habits	15
41	Vacation	13
42	Christmas	12
43	Minor violations of the law	11

Here is a good way to learn to breathe with your diaphragm:

♦ Find a quiet, comfortable place to sit or lie down.
♦ Place your feet slightly apart. Place one hand on your naval and the other hand on your chest.
♦ Inhale through your nose and exhale through your mouth.
♦ Concentrate on your breathing by noticing which hand is rising and falling with each breath.
♦ Gently exhale most of the air in your lungs.
♦ Inhale while slowly counting to 4. As you inhale, slightly extend your abdomen, causing it to rise about 1 (1) inch. Make sure you are not moving your chest or shoulders.
♦ As you breath in, imagine the warmed air flowing in and going into all parts of your body.
♦ Pause for one (1) second then slowly exhale to the count of 4. As you exhale, your abdomen should move inward.
♦ As the air flows out, imagine all your tensions and stress leaving your body.
♦ Repeat the process until you achieve a sense of deep relaxation.

Progressive relaxation is the act of contracting one muscle group at a time, holding it in contraction, then relaxing the muscles. Begin by contracting the muscles of your face and neck, holding the contraction for a period of at least 2 seconds, and then relax the muscles. Next contract and relax your upper arms and chest, followed by your lower arms and hands. Repeat the process progressively down your body: abdomen, buttocks, thighs, calves, and feet. Then repeat the whole sequence two or three times.

See your medical doctor when...

- You have uncontrollable anger and do not know why.
- You have insomnia.
- You have difficulty sustaining relationships.
- You have persistent feelings of guilt.
- You consistently rehash incidents in your mind.

Mental:

Imagery - Imagine you are in a different place or situation than you are at the moment stress begins to take over. See yourself moving away from a bad moment and moving into a very tranquil place. Do this while deep breathing and music playing. It is important to stay as focused as possible.

Positive Affirmation – Write down all the things you would like to change or to have happen in your life as if they have already happened. Say these every day during your quiet time. You will see these things for which you have affirmed actually take place. This is so positive. as it puts you there mentally before you get there physically. What the mind thinks will happen.

Practice Positive Thinking – Talk to yourself when negative thinking begins to envelope you. Go to a mirror; look at yourself while you are talking to yourself. This will put you in touch with yourself. Think of all the things you have instead of the things you do not have.

Read Self-Help Books – There are so many books that can help us get through troubling times. It just means getting to the local bookstore to find what you need. You might also find someone very interesting with whom you can share a conversation over a cup of coffee.

Music Therapy – Settles the mind and body. There are also CDs and tapes on meditation that focus on color, sounds and music. Deep breathing while listening to this music is very healing.

Flower and Herbal Therapy – Several ingredients within the flower and herb family are very conducive to relaxation. Perhaps because of their vibrant colors or their lovely fragrances, flowers seem to have a therapeutic effect when we are fighting illness, fatigue, or flagging spirits. Herbs have long been used as medicinal remedies. Essential oils are products of either flowers or herbs and play a very important part in skin care and healing essences.

Reflexology – The feet and hands have corresponding areas that are associated with other parts of the body. If that part of the hand or foot is massaged, there is usually relief in the corresponding part of the body. Special attention is paid to those areas, which have correlation to the spine, pituitary, thyroid, parathyroid, adrenal glands, and the diaphragm. *Aromatherapy* - The use of flower and herbal therapy is usually as an inhalant. It can also be used topically and in some cases can be ingested.

Intellectual:

♦ Read at least one book each week on a subject that most interests you.
♦ Attend seminars.
♦ Attend classes at a local college or university.
♦ Find ways to increase your knowledge.

Social:

♦ Set up a support system: family, friends, clergy, support group, and working peers. It is said that a person survives best with more than 6 people they can count on to "be there" in times of need.
♦ Attend cultural events.
♦ Attend social events.
♦ Investigate the services/program at a workout gym.
♦ Attend athletic events.
♦ Take dancing lessons.

Spiritual:

♦ Set aside one hour each day to meditate. This could be thinking about nature, a higher power, or anything beautiful around you.
♦ Get some meditation books – these will help you stay focused.
♦ Get OK with life and how you feel about eternity. All of us are *terminal* – we will not get out of this world alive.
♦ Each day be grateful for five things you have, e.g., good health, great job, working automobile, roof over your head, etc.
♦ Read one chapter/verse of the Bible or a spiritual book each day.

- Attend a spiritual study group or meditate regularly.
- Pray for those who have offended you.
- ***Love*** and ***Forgive*** **yourself and others.**
- Bring in all the "Light" you can, and then let it shine for others to see – ***Let Your Light Shine***!
- Keep in your prayers all those suffering from debilitating diseases.

Chapter 10

Miscellaneous
Information

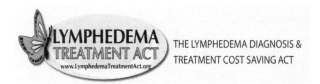

THE LYMPHEDEMA DIAGNOSIS &
TREATMENT COST SAVING ACT

Overview:

The Lymphedema Treatment Act would offer coverage for Medicare beneficiaries with lymphedema from any cause. It would provide the medically recommended protocols (compression bandages, garments, and supplies used daily in the treatment and management of lymphedema) and reduce the incidence of lymphedema-related infection. Although this legislation relates specifically to a change in Medicare law, it would also have the almost certain effect of ensuring all private insurance policies follow suit.

Lymphedema is a medial condition which results in a swelling of any part of the body when the lymphatic vessels and/or lymph nodes are damaged or are inadequate. Lymphedema affects an estimate 1.5 to 3 million Medicare beneficiaries who currently receive sub-standard treatment from Medicare according to the current medical standard of care. Medicare is spending hundreds of millions of dollars every year in hospitalizations for largely preventable lymphedema-related Cellulitis.

Bill Goals:

- to provide diagnosis and treatment of individuals with and at risk for lymphedema according to current medical treatment standards, including manual lymph drainage, compression bandages, garments, devices, and exercise;
- to provide for lymphedema patient education in the procedures for self-treatment so as to transfer the treatment from the clinical to the home setting;
- to encourage patient self-treatment plan adherence by providing necessary medical supplies for use at home;
- to reduce total healthcare costs through avoidance of periodic infections, pain, and disabilities resulting from this medical condition.

This bill is projected to save hundreds of millions of dollars every year in avoidance of costs of treating preventable lymphedema-related cellulitis. This is a quality of care issue affecting insured patients and is complementary to healthcare access issues.

What you can do:

Please contact your members of Congress by using the submission forms at the www.LymphedemaTreatmentAct.org website. There you will also find many other simple ways you can support the passage of this bill and ensure that lymphedema sufferers get the medically necessary treatment coverage they need and deserve.

For more information about the Lymphedema Treatment Act:
www.LymphedemaTreatmentAct.org | info@LymphedemaTreatmentAct.org

For more information about Lymphedema and its Treatment visit:
National Lymphedema Network | www.lymphnet.org | NLN@lymphnet.org | (415) 908-3681

Anatomy of the Breast

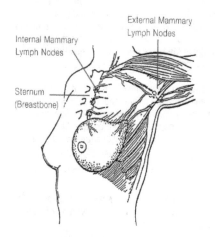

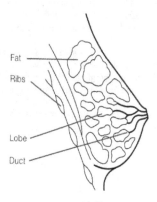

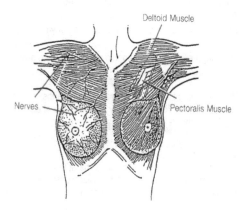

Breast Self-Exam

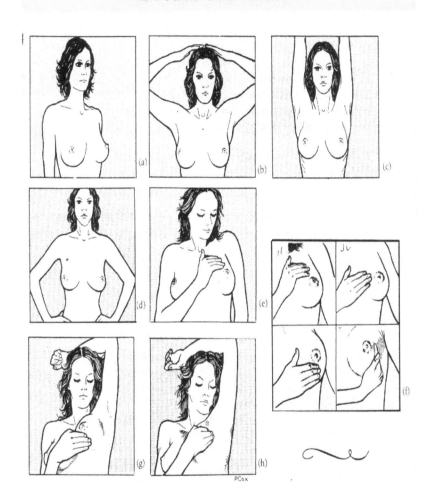

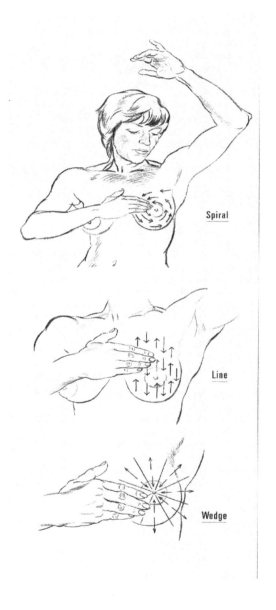

Spiral

Line

Wedge

141

Guide to Proper Fitting Post-Mastectomy

◆ Fit existing breast into appropriate bra size.

◆ Check bra/prosthesis sizing chart for correct prosthesis size.

◆ Place prosthesis into prosthesis cover and place inside mastectomy bra pocket on affected side.

◆ While you are wearing bra with prosthesis inside bra pocket:

- Stand in front of mirror to visually test for breast symmetry, size, and if both breasts appear even, vertically and horizontally.

- Look down at breasts checking to see if they protrude out equally from the torso – top view.

- Turn from side to side, right and left, checking to see if breasts extend out equally from the torso – side view.

- While you are wearing bra with prosthesis, feel both breasts to see if they feel very nearly the same size and proportion inside bra cups.

- Check weight – seeing if weight of both breasts is proportioned equally between bra straps and bra band.

- Check body balance – Do you feel balanced with new prosthesis inserted? Do both breasts feel the same weight? Does the prosthesis equalize upper body weight?

- Check bulging of breast tissue either in axilla or upper chest above bra. If this is the case, the bra cups are too small. Try either a larger cup size or go up in a band size, e.g., 34B to 36A, or 34B to 34C.

- **Note:** As band size increases, cup size decreases.

Final test — Overall, how do you feel?
- Raise both arms.
- Sit down.
- Take a deep breath.
- Put on a shirt/blouse.
- Check to see if you have a natural look that is void of bra-cup puckering, undesirable seams, and/or wrong bra color.

Eating During Cancer Treatment:

- Patients who eat well during treatment are able to cope better with the side effects of treatment.
- Patients who eat well may be able to handle a higher dose of their treatment.
- A nutritious diet will keep your strength up, prevent catabolism of body tissue, and promote rebuilding of tissue that cancer treatment may break down.

It is important to consume a diet containing a variety of different food everyday to keep your body strong:

- **Fruits & Vegetables** – provides certain vitamins and minerals the body needs.
- **Protein** – fights infection and assists in your body's healing process. Contains many vitamins and minerals.
- **Grains & Starch** – provides a good source of energy for the body to perform well.
- **Dairy** – provide many vitamins and protein.

Keep a variety of snacks around to improve your nutrition to lessen the side effects of your treatment and to keep your food intake up.

Here are some quick snack ideas to have in stock:

Applesauce	Bread products (muffins & crackers)
Granola	Gelatin salads & desserts
Buttered popcorn	Hard-boiled & deviled eggs
Fruits	Ice cream, frozen yogurt, & popsicles
Cereal	Milkshakes, instant breakfast drinks
Nuts	Cheese, hard or semisoft
Peanut butter	Cheesecake
Pizza	Chocolate milk
Cottage cheese	Quesadillas
Sandwiches	Cream cheese & other soft cheese
Cream soups	Vegetables

Yogurt (regular or frozen)
Puddings & custards
Dips made with cheese, beans, or sour cream
Dried fruits, such as raisins, prunes, or apricots
Cakes & cookies made with whole-grains, fruits, nuts, wheat
germ, or granola

Once your treatment begins, your body will need plenty of rest and sustenance to keep your nutrition up. Here are some useful suggestions:

♦ When possible, let someone else cook your meals.

♦ As you get more familiar with your recovery time after treatment, have someone help out with shopping, cooking, and cleaning.

♦ Choose meals that you and your family can "throw together" easily. Cook large batches to freeze for future meals.

♦ Have written instructions available so other may help out.

♦ When making casseroles for freezing, only partially cook items such as rice and macaroni. They will cook some more when you reheat them.

♦ When people offer to help out, whether it be cooking meals or shopping, let them.

♦ Use mixes, ready-to-eat meals, and takeout to decrease time spent on cooking and cleaning, and more time to relax and spend time with your family.

Neutropenic Diet

Neutropenia is a condition caused by having a low white blood cell count, causing a suppressed immune system. A person low in neutropenics is more prone to develop an infection. Infections like these can be caused by bacteria found in food and beverages.

Review the following dietary guidelines to help reduce your risk for infection.

Foods to *Avoid*:

- All fresh or dried fruits & vegetables, including garnishes

- Raw or rare-cooked meats, fish, or eggs

- Unpasteurized dairy products (i.e.. raw milk, naturally aged cheeses, and yogurt)

- Cheeses with mold or soft cheeses

- Fresh herbs & seasonings (unless they are added during cooking)

- Cold cuts and processed meats (hot dogs, ham, bologna, salami, sausage) that are not commercially packaged

- Shellfish

- Fresh salad dressings containing aged cheeses

- Unpasteurized apple cider, eggnog, homemade lemonade, spring water

- Raw honey

- Foods from street vendors, salad bars, coffee carts, delis; or beverages that are not prepackaged

Choose the following foods in individual containers to reduce the possibility of bacteria–induced infection:

- Juice
- Bread
- Margarine or butter
- Jelly
- Pasteurized milk & milk products
- Creamer
- Sugar or sugar substitute
- Ice cream, commercial pastries, frozen yogurt, sherbet, ice cream bars
- Canned or frozen fruits or vegetables
- Commercially packaged luncheon meats

It is extremely important to practice proper food handling and preparation to prevent bacterial growth.

Care of Bandages

♦ All bandages touching the skin (tubular, short or long-stretch, stockinette & finger bandages) should be washed daily. Short stretch, long stretch, padding, and pressure pieces not in contact with the skin can be washed every 3 days – more frequently in warm weather and/or if soiled. All the above except foam is washable.

♦ Wash all bandages in tepid water using a mild liquid soap such as *Ivory* or *Dreft* – **No *Woolite* & no soap powders.**

♦ Place bandages in a lingerie bag before putting in washing machine. Wash on slow cycle, fast spin.

♦ Dry bandages on a flat surface, hang them over a drying rack, or over a shower stall. Roll them tightly after they are dry.

♦ Avoid ironing bandages or cutting them.

♦ Roll bandages immediately after removing them from the bandaged arm or leg.

♦ Do not use "clips" to fasten bandages – use tape to secure bandages in place.

♦ If using bandages daily, they need to be replaced every 2 -3 months.

Care of Garments

- Compression garments are washed in tepid water every day after wear, using a mild liquid detergent such as *Ivory* or *Dreft* — **No *Woolite* & no soap powders.**
- **Wash inside out.**
- Rinse garment thoroughly in tepid water & squeeze out excess water – do not twist or wring.
- Roll garment in thick fluffy towel to get all excess water out – hang to dry overnight.
- Purchase at least 2 garments – wear one while the other is laundered.
- **Never sleep in gradient compression garments.**
- If you are wearing one garment daily, it will maintain its compression for approximately 3 months — replace every 3-4 months.
- Purchase a new garment before the old one has lost its compression.
- Before applying garment first time, put the day's date on inside band with an indelible pen.
- Apply garments with rubber gloves to avoid any ripping or snagging – making sure weave of fabric is even up the limb.
- Do not overstretch the garment when applying it.
- **Make sure weave of garment is smoothed out from end to end.**

Care of
Farrow Wraps

Wash *Farrow Wraps* once a week or if soiled.

♦ *Farrow Wraps* are washed in a sink or tub in tepid water once a week, using a mild liquid detergent such as *Ivory* or *Dreft*. **No *Woolite* — no soap powder.**

♦ After washing, rinse garment thoroughly in tepid water & squeeze out excess water – do not twist or wring.

♦ Roll *Farrow Wraps* in thick fluffy towel to remove any excess water.

♦ Dry flat on a towel or an open rack.

♦ Purchase at least 2 *Farrow Wraps* – wear one while the other is in reserve.

♦ **If you are wearing a *Farrow Wrap* daily, it will maintain its compression & stretch for approximately 6-8 months – replace every 6-8 months.**

♦ Purchase a new *Farrow Wrap* before the old one has lost compression and/or stretch.

♦ Before applying *Farrow Wrap* the first time, put the day's date on inside band with an indelible pen.

♦ Tighten straps beginning at ankle and continue to below knee and close with Velcro strips.

♦ *Farrow Wraps* must be applied gradiently – most compression at the ankle with decreasing compression ascending the leg.

♦ Do not overstretch straps when applying the *Farrow Wrap*.

♦ Goal of *Farrow Wraps* is to reduce swelling and pain, increase mobility and protect wound healing environment.

♦ The *Farrow Wrap* is either Classic or Strong-Trim-To-Fit and is 30-40mmHg (CCL-2) pressure beginning at the ankle. If reduction takes place, you may need to trim the straps.

New *Custom* Gradient Compression Garments

Lymphedema is constantly changing.

♦ From the time of measuring until fitting, circumference of the affected body part will be different from when it was at the time of measuring.
♦ Flat knit fabric, designed for custom garments, must be "unforgiving" so that the swelling of the affected area is contained.
♦ When custom garments arrive, approximately 10-14 days following measure/order, fitting takes place and instructions in daily care of garments is given.
♦ Because flat knit fabric is unforgiving and designed to contain swelling, the fabric as well as the surged seams need time to relax. It is necessary to build up time wearing custom garments and follow the fitter's instructions. This will help relax surged seams and fabric.
♦ In the case of custom gloves, wash the garment per instructions and, while the garment is still moist, insert "sharpie" highlighter pens into the fingers to loosen the fabric and the surged seams. Leave in overnight while the garment is not being worn.

Remember: When wearing gradient compression garments for the first time, tissues of the affected area are not familiar with gradient compression, and they will react. So, be patient and build up time wearing them gradually.

Hand & Foot
Intensive Therapy

♦ Wash hands/feet — rinse well.

♦ While skin/nails are still moist, apply A&D
Ointment all over and work in well.

Mix A&D Ointment with following essential oils:
Lavender
Tea Tree
Eucalyptus
Lemon
or
Peppermint

Ratio = 3-5 drops essential oil to a
tablespoon of A&D ointment or lotion

♦ Massage in very well.

♦ Apply gloves on hands and stockings for feet.

♦ **Sleep with application all night.**

Appendix

Definitions

Bilateral – both sides of the body or both extremities, e,g., Both arms, both legs.

Cellulitis – a diffuse, acute infection of the skin and subcutaneous tissue characterized most commonly by heat, redness, pain, swelling in an affected body part or area. Occasionally there is generalized fever, discomfort, chills, and headache.

Circumferential – measuring around a body part

CDT – Combined Decongestive Therapy

Depilatory – ingredient that removes body hair

Distal – away from or being the farthest from a point of origin. Example: the hands are distal to the shoulder and torso

Embolism – a blood clot traveling in the bloodstream

Exfoliate – remove dead cells and debris from the surface of the skin

Elephantiasis – tremendous swelling with overlying skin becoming dark, thick and coarse, similar to elephant skin

Gradient Pressure – most pressure at the farthest point, gradually decreasing to the nearest point of an extremity

DFG – Directional Flow Garment

Fibrosis – hardening/thickening of the tissues

Fibrous – threadlike, woodsy

Hemangioma – a benign tumor consisting of a mass of blood vessels

Intercellular – between cells

Invasive – anything that intrudes upon the body

Klippel-Trenaunay Syndrome – congenital condition affecting bones, blood vessels, and body tissues with manifestations of port-wine stains on the skin

Leprosy – a disease that affects the skin and other tissues of the body, causing decay

Lymph – the fluid that originates in the spaces between body cells

Lymphatic – lymph vessel carrying lymph

Lymphangioma – congenital, benign, often cystic malformations of the lymphatics

Lymph Node – (see *Introduction, p. 13*)

Lymphocyte – a disease-fighting white blood cell

mmHg – millimeters of Mercury pressure, used in thermometers, barometers, and other measuring instruments

Macrophage – a killing white blood cell

MLD – Manual Lymph Drainage

Peripheral Lymphatic Vessel – lymphatic vessels near the surface of the body, just under the skin

Proximal – nearer to a point of reference, the closest point Example: the ear is proximal to the head.

Self MLD – Self Manual Lymph Drainage

Sequential – happening in succession, as in pump chambers inflating and deflating in succession from farthest point (distal) to nearest point (proximal)

Seroma – a pocket or cystic sac in which there is a collection of blood and lymph fluids, usually appears near an incision area following surgery

Supinate (Supine) – lying on the back with face up, palm of hand facing up ("Sup is Up")

Thrombophlebitis – inflammation of a vein with a blood clot

Thrombosis – a blood clot in a vein

Unilateral – one side of the body or one extremity

Index

About the Author

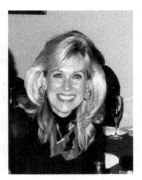

Phyllis Tubbs-Gingerich holds a diploma and a BS in nursing with a specialty in skin, wound care, lymphedema and cancer care. She has been a Vodder/LANA certified lymphedema therapist for 30+ years, and has over 40 years' experience in cancer care.

As a memorial to her sister, Maria, Phyllis established the Ginger-K Center in San Jose, CA in 1989. It is dedicated to anyone needing care and support following diagnosis of cancer and the effects of lymphedema.

Phyllis' focus is to give patients knowledge and insight into their medical conditions so that they can develop the courage to care for themselves and make wise decisions about their health and well-being.

When it became apparent that more information and education about lymphedema was necessary and patients needed a source to give, receive and share this information, Phyllis founded the Lymphedema Information Support Group (LISG) in 1997.

LISG sponsored the 1st Lymphedema Care Forum on June 8, 2001, in Morgan Hill, CA. A huge success, over 250 physicians, nurses, patients, and their families attended. The 2nd, 3rd, and 4th Lymphedema Care Forums were held, again in Morgan Hill, in October 2003, October 2005, and June 2012, respectively.

LISG became a state and federal nonprofit organization in 2002. Its purpose is to be a resource for education and information about lymphedema, and to assist in financially supporting lymphedema care for those who otherwise cannot afford it, especially children with primary lymphedema.

In order to teach other professional care-givers how to care for patients with lymphedema, Ginger-K Center received credentialing in 2002 from the California Board of Registered Nursing to provide continuing education for medical professionals.

In preparation for lymphedema care becoming a medical specialty, Phyllis has created an Internship Program for high school and college students seeking medical careers to interest them in one day becoming MD Lymphedema Specialists. She also teaches an advanced practicum and apprenticeship course to lymphedema therapists wanting to "bone up on their skills."

Phyllis has created a series of power point presentations instructing people in better self-care, so as to reduce the incidences of cancer and other chronic debilitating diseases.

Ginger-K Lymphedema & Cancer Care Center
16275 Monterey Rd,
Classic Square, Suite E
Morgan Hill, CA 95037-5527
www.gingerkcenter.com
phyllis@gingerkcenter.com
Phone: (408) 782-1028
Fax: (408) 782-1061

Coming soon by Phyllis: *One Journey Around The Sun*

CPSIA information can be obtained
at www.ICGtesting.com
Printed in the USA
JSHW031455220123
36478JS00005B/21

9 780615 634210